The Resilient Nurse:
Empowering Your Practice

Margaret McAllister, RN, MHN, BA (UQ), MEd (ACU), EdD (QUT), is a professor of nursing at the University of the Sunshine Coast, Maroochydore, Australia. A fellow of the Australian College of Mental Health Nursing and of the Royal College of Nursing, Australia, a credentialed mental health nurse and registered nurse, she is widely published in nursing internationally. Her innovative concept, "Solution Focused Nursing," is the theme of her 2007 book *Solution Focused Nursing: Rethinking Practice* (London: Macmillan-Palgrave). In 2010, McAllister was honoured to receive an Australian Learning and Teaching Council Citation for the development of this innovative concept as an effective way of developing high-level caring skills in nurses.

As well as coordinating the Master of Mental Health Nursing, Margaret is the director of the Australian Collaborative for Transformational Learning in Health—a group that aims to work across disciplines to promote educational excellence. She supervises several higher degree students in nursing research projects. She is currently involved in six collaborative research projects: They range from exploring nursing history, evaluating a school nursing intervention around self-harm, mental health leadership, and the future of nursing. She has published more than 100 book chapters and journal articles.

John B. Lowe, BSc, MPH, DrPH, is a professor and head of the School of Health and Sport Sciences at the University of the Sunshine Coast, Australia, where he holds the chair in Population Health. He is a fellow of the Australian Health Promotion Association and the American Academy of Health Behavior. Dr. Lowe is currently the senior editor of the *Australian and New Zealand Journal of Public Health* and was previously the editor of *Health Promotion Journal of Australia*. Previous posts include professor and head, Department of Community and Behavioural Health, College of Public Health, University of Iowa; associate director for Population Science, Holden Comprehensive Cancer Center, University of Iowa; and director, Cancer Prevention Research Centre at the University of Queensland. He was the principal investigator on 13 U.S. grants, two of seven figures, seven of six figures. He is the main or coauthor on 145 peer-reviewed publications. He continues to focus his research on community development and empowerment to make sustainable long-term changes to promote health. He is a graduate of the University of Texas Health Science Center, School of Public Health.

The Resilient Nurse: Empowering Your Practice

Margaret McAllister, RN, MHN, BA, MEd, EdD

John B. Lowe, BSc, MPH, DrPH

Editors

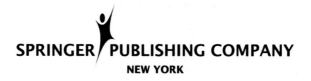

SPRINGER PUBLISHING COMPANY
NEW YORK

Copyright © 2011 Springer Publishing Company, LLC

Springer Publishing Company, LLC
11 West 42nd Street
New York, NY 10036
www.springerpub.com

Acquisitions Editor: Allan Graubard
Senior Editor: Rose Mary Piscitelli
Cover design: Joseph DePinho
Project Manager: Gil Rafanan
Composition: Absolute Service, Inc.

ISBN: 978-0-8261-0593-6
E-book ISBN: 978-0-8261-0594-3

12 13 14/ 5 4 3 2

The author and the publisher of this Work have made every effort to use sources believed to be reliable to provide information that is accurate and compatible with the standards generally accepted at the time of publication. Because medical science is continually advancing, our knowledge base continues to expand. Therefore, as new information becomes available, changes in procedures become necessary. We recommend that the reader always consult current research and specific institutional policies before performing any clinical procedure. The author and publisher shall not be liable for any special, consequential, or exemplary damages resulting, in whole or in part, from the readers' use of, or reliance on, the information contained in this book. The publisher has no responsibility for the persistence or accuracy of URLs for external or third-party Internet websites referred to in this publication and does not guarantee that any content on such Web sites is, or will remain, accurate or appropriate.

CIP data is available from the Library of Congress

Special discounts on bulk quantities of our books are available to corporations, professional associations, pharmaceutical companies, health care organizations, and other qualifying groups.

If you are interested in a custom book, including chapters from more than one of our titles, we can provide that service as well.

For details, please contact:
Special Sales Department, Springer Publishing Company, LLC
11 West 42nd Street, 15th Floor, New York, NY 10036-8002
Phone: 877-687-7476 or 212-431-4370; Fax: 212-941-7842
Email: sales@springerpub.com

Printed in the United States of America by Gasch Printing

To the many nurses who are inspirations to us all

Contents

Contributors   ix
Foreword   xi
Preface   xiii
Acknowledgment   xvii

1. Preparing for Practice: Becoming Resilient   *1*
   Margaret McAllister and John B. Lowe

2. Nurses Who Made a Difference   *23*
   Margaret McAllister and John B. Lowe

3. Moral and Ethical Practice   *31*
   Andrew Estefan

4. Learning From Role Models   *43*
   Maura MacPhee

5. Thinking Clearly: Realistic Appraisals and
   Moderating Reactions in Stressful Situations   *59*
   Mary Katsikitis and Rachael R. Sharman

6. Being Convincing: Talking to Others Persuasively   *75*
   *Natoshia M. Askelson, Mary Lober Aquilino,
   and Shelly Campo*

7. Mind Games at Work: Preparing for Effective Team-Working   *91*
   Tony Warne and Sue McAndrew

8. Thriving in the Workplace:
   Learning From Innovative Practices   *105*
   *Debra Jackson, Glenda McDonald,
   and Lesley Wilkes*

9. What to Do When the Busy Day Is Over   *115*
   *Jane Brannan, Mary de Chesnay,
   and Patricia L. Hart*

10. Things Just Got Really Serious: Coping in Crisis   *133*
    Jane Shakespeare-Finch

11. Now It's My Turn: Becoming the Image of the Good Leader   *149*
    Linda Shields

12. Looking Forward   *167*
    Margaret McAllister and John B. Lowe

Index   *173*

Contributors

Mary Lober Aquilino, MSN, PhD, FNP   Assistant Dean and Master of Public Health Program Director, Associate Professor (Community and Behavioral Health), College of Public Health, University of Iowa, Iowa City, IA

Natoshia M. Askelson, MPH, PhD   Assistant Research Scientist, Assistant Director, Center for Health Communication and Social Marketing, College of Public Health, University of Iowa, Iowa City, IA

Jane Brannan, EdD, RN   Associate Professor and Assistant Director (Undergraduate Nursing), WellStar School of Nursing, Kennesaw State University, Kennesaw, GA

Shelly Campo, PhD   Associate Professor, Director, Center for Health Communication and Social Marketing, College of Public Health, University of Iowa, Iowa City, IA

Mary de Chesnay, DSN, RN, PMHCNS-BC, FAAN   Director, WellStar School of Nursing, Kennesaw State University, Kennesaw, GA

Andrew Estefan, RPN, DipNSc, BN, MN, PhD   Assistant Professor, Faculty of Nursing, University of Calgary, Calgary, Canada

Patricia L. Hart, RN, PhD   Assistant Professor (Nursing), Kennesaw State University, Kennesaw, GA

Debra Jackson, RN, PhD   Family and Community Health Research Group (FaCH), School of Nursing and Midwifery, College of Health and Science, University of Western Sydney, Sydney, NSW, Australia

Mary Katsikitis, PhD   Professor (Psychology), Faculty of Arts and Social Sciences, University of the Sunshine Coast, Maroochydore DC, QLD, Australia

John B. Lowe, BSc, MPH, DrPH   Head of School, School of Health and Sport Sciences, Professor (Population Health Sciences), Faculty of Science, Health and Education, University of the Sunshine Coast, Maroochydore DC, QLD, Australia

Maura MacPhee, RN, PhD   Assistant Professor, School of Nursing, University of British Columbia, Vancouver, BC, Canada

Margaret McAllister, RN, MHN, BA, MEd, EdD   Professor of Nursing, School of Health and Sport Sciences, Faculty of Science, Health and Education, University of the Sunshine Coast, Maroochydore DC, QLD, Australia

Sue McAndrew, RMN, CPN Cert, BSc (Hons), MSc, PhD   Research Fellow (Mental Health), School of Nursing and Midwifery, University of Salford, Greater Manchester, United Kingdom

Glenda McDonald, BSocSc, GradDipSocSc (Adult Ed)   Doctoral Student, PhD candidate Nursing, Family and Community Health Research Group (FaCH), School of Nursing and Midwifery, College of Health and Science, University of Western Sydney, Sydney, NSW, Australia

Jane Shakespeare-Finch, PhD   Senior Lecturer, School of Psychology and Counselling, School of Psychology and Counselling, Faculty of Health, Queensland University of Technology, Kelvin Grove, QLD, Australia

Rachael R. Sharman, BA, BPsych (Hons)   Research Assistant, Psychology, Faculty of Arts and Social Sciences, University of the Sunshine Coast, Maroochydore DC, QLD, Australia

Linda Shields, BAppSci (Nursing), MMedSci, PhD, FRCNA, FRSM   Professor (Paediatric and Child Health Nursing), School of Nursing and Midwifery, Curtin University, and Child and Adolescent Health Service, Perth, WA, Honorary Professor (Paediatrics and Child Health), University of Queensland, Australia

Tony Warne, PhD, MBA, RMN   Head of School, School of Nursing and Midwifery, Professor (Mental Health Care), University of Salford, Greater Manchester, United Kingdom

Lesley Wilkes, PhD, RN   Professor (Nursing) and Research Coordinator, School of Nursing and Midwifery, University of Western Sydney, Penrith, NSW, Australia

Foreword

Although most nurses find their careers rewarding, many would also agree that they work in a profession that not only is physically and psychologically challenging but is also not always as nurturing as you would expect. In this book, the authors have created a rich resource to provide support for nurses and students of nursing in developing the resilience they need to cope with these challenges.

Few people outside of the health professions would easily recognise that healing work can be personally taxing. With such a drain on energy, it is often easier to be self-protective to the extent that we are not able to support others. Using the strategies from this book, we can find better ways to care for ourselves, our colleagues, and, therefore, our clients.

The authors use case studies, storytelling, and reflective learning exercises judiciously throughout the book to make the strategies for increasing resilience accessible to nurses at all stages of their professional careers. With these guides, we can better prepare nurses for the realities of practice and, by doing so, ultimately change the culture of nursing.

The concept of resilience, and how to foster it, underpins the authors' purpose for this book. More than courage, and different from endurance, resilience is a quality we find worthy of admiration. To describe someone as resilient implies not only that he or she has survived adversity, but also that he or she has learnt from the experience and developed personally because of it.

The value of this book lies in the concept that resilience is not necessarily something that only the lucky and genetically endowed few attain. Yes, there are some personal characteristics that no doubt make some people likely to be more resilient than others—having empathy and being intuitive and adaptable, for example. However, people can learn to seek or to create certain things in their lives that promote resilience; things like good friendships and loving relationships, or practising to express their feelings more honestly, or working at responding to negative experiences in ways that do not exacerbate the situation. Employing the many strategies brought together in this text should enable individuals to increase their caring for colleagues and for themselves and, by these seemingly simple changes, bring about cultural change in the profession.

This is a practical guide that is nevertheless firmly grounded in evidence. The theory underpinning the proposed strategies is well described, and knowledge about how children and adults deal with hardship is applied to various approaches for dealing with the rigours of nursing. Additionally, the techniques help to cope with the questionable practices of colleagues who create hardship for others by their behaviour and actions. With the tools from this book, nurses should be able to survive and thrive, and gain the strength and tactics to break the cycles of hostility and workplace negativity, and thereby change the system.

The totality of the book is greater than the sum of its chapters. The authors of each of the 12 chapters have taken a different perspective on the issue, and so provided a range of tools for increasing resilience, providing support, and learning optimism. For those who are not naturally resilient, this book provides coaching and lessons in setting goals and elevating their expectations. The authors have also provided many role models of nurses who have demonstrated the leadership and tenacity that guides others to develop their own self-confidence and to not only face but also overcome adversity.

If we are lucky, we may never face real adversity in our lives, and may therefore never become aware of our capacity to emerge with new strength and knowledge about ourselves. However, if we learn the lessons provided in this book, we should develop the self-understanding and skills necessary to find meaning in experiences that are not optimal and to moderate our own reactions to the stresses of daily work in imperfect environments.

Through finding good mentors, using humour, enjoying pets, meditating, exercising, and self-reflecting—just some among the many suggested strategies in this book—we should reach the stage of being able to deal with the realities of nursing through either changing the situation or changing our own interpretations of, and reactions to, that situation. With greater support for and from colleagues, we can focus on ameliorating the stresses intrinsic to healing work. When our emotions are invested in our patients and clients, completely eliminating stress is impossible (and probably undesirable). However, through using the strategies provided in this book, we should all be able to cope with the traumas of everyday nursing practice with more grace and resilience than before.

Stephanie Fox-Young, RN, PhD, FRCNA
Associate Professor
President of the Royal College of Nursing, Australia

Preface

As a reader and a student of nursing, you are in a fortunate position. Unlike many of your predecessors who underwent "learn-on-the-job" training, you now have the opportunity to explore common cultural and social problems encountered in health care from the relative safety of your own armchair or classroom. You do not necessarily have to experience these problems to learn from them.

Think about how your first day of being a nurse might be. Now, imagine if it went like this: The first person you see as you enter the nurses' station is the team leader and she does not look happy. "Oh, hello there," she greets, with an unmistakable undertone of sarcasm that you've heard several times before, but in your student days. You thought that kind of attitude was in the past. Your bright and expectant smile begins to fade.

"A brand new graduate! Just what we need today. Oh well, time to get you sorted then. I hope you've got your running shoes on because we are down two nurses today so you're going to have to take seven clients instead of four. And, because I'm feeling extra nice today, I'm allocating you Mrs. Hanson. She's heading for a respiratory arrest, the night staff tells me, so I think that would be perfect for you. Jump right into the deep end. You've also got Jonesy. He's a real trick. You'll find out what I mean. Now, get into the handover. Being late is not a good look. Oh and by the way, welcome to the real world!"

As you head home later, you realise that you have three choices: (a) you can listen to that little voice and go home, decide it's all too much, jump on the Internet and look for a new job; (b) you can go back tomorrow, determined to fit in by modelling yourself closely on the team leader's words and actions; or (c) you can reflect on what you've learned from this book and realise that you have other choices, strategies, and resiliency skills to practise nursing according to your own values and beliefs. The challenge, now, is that you just need to apply them.

Within this book, several workplace challenges are discussed. You will read about strategies to avoid or resolve such challenges. In this way, you are going to be more prepared for difficult encounters. In a sense, you will be inoculated against events that might otherwise be shocking, frustrating, or overwhelming. Rather than feeling powerless, you can arm yourself with awareness and problem-solving strategies to help you feel powerful and more confident about being a positive influence. As a result, you're likely to feel less self-doubt, less tentativeness, and less emotional distress.

The aim of this book is to inspire you to develop your capabilities so that you become a strong, determined, enthusiastic, and effective clinician, even in the face of challenges, hardships, and disappointment. These challenges will come, make no mistake; the health care world isn't perfect. You will encounter sadness, pain, worry, impatience, frustration, and conflict. There will be real ethical dilemmas in which the choices you face are equally valid, and you will have to make heart-rending decisions. There will be mistakes and some of these will be yours. There will be times when you are frightened, outside of your comfort zone and not able to retreat. And there may even come a time when you begin to question, as we all do, your own effectiveness—*If what I'm doing makes a difference, then why is it that people continue to suffer?*

However, if you cultivate the qualities and use the strategies revealed in this book, your "existential despair" will be short-lived and renewed determination will emerge. For in the scheme of things, nurses have shown time and time again that they are a precious and vital resource for society. We are the hand that reaches out to offer comfort and connection. We are the voice that translates jargon into understanding. We are the actors that transform crisis into coping. We are, and ought to be, the leaders in advancing the human face of health care. Moreover, we are not alone in this endeavour. Every other clinician working alongside us is charged with the same responsibility to move beyond the technique, the clipboard, and the machinery to be a better human being. Although other clinicians have their specific skills and focuses, nurses are the lynchpins of health services. Nurses are the human face of health services, for when people think of hospitals, they think of nurses. When people think of care, they think of nurses. Therefore, when things go wrong in health care, when people are dehumanised or experience undue suffering, people look to nurses, the surrogate mother or father, to look out for them, to take charge, and to bring back order and control. Thus, our place in the health care environment, individually and collectively, is not only important, it is formative in shaping the landscape.

Gandhi, the Indian philosopher and leader, once famously said, "Be the change you want to see in the world." His message was simple, yet profound. What does it mean to you? Perhaps he was stressing the importance of living your life in ways that will make a positive difference. Furthermore, it may mean that our working life may contain challenges that we don't have to just endure. Rather, we can change our circumstances by having the courage to act in ways that may not be popular, but are true to our values and our hopes. That's how Gandhi lived his life. He chose to object (thoughtfully and carefully) to injustice. He thought actions were more powerful than words, but he used both to great effect. He was an orator and a role model. He experienced personal conflict and pain, but believed in active peacemaking for the benefit of the world. His enduring message, applied to nursing, is that what you do *can* make a difference, not only to the individual clients whose lives you touch but also to the entire health care service. You will influence people both directly and indirectly. People will watch you and learn from you; their lives may be transformed by a single encounter with you. It will not be easy and you won't be a leader at the very beginning, but with determination and some words of inspiration found, we hope, within the pages of this book, the personal qualities that led you to nursing will develop into mature leadership skills.

This book is structured in sections that will help you to develop resilience and to be empowered to make changes based on thought rather than on reaction. You may, in your own life, have already developed many of the skills required, and the chapters will be a booster shot to continue to develop your abilities:

Chapter 1 introduces the concept of resilience for practice in the health professions.

Chapter 2 considers the qualities of two nursing leaders who made an enduring difference to the world and, of course, to nursing.

Chapter 3 looks at ethical thinking to help us appraise and then to think through dilemmas that could otherwise cause distress.

Chapter 4 discusses the empowerment that can be achieved through the conscious observation of positive role models.

Chapter 5 focuses on the thought processes that can assist us to think more positively about challenges that may present.

Chapter 6 explores communication theories that explain some of the sources of misunderstandings in the workplace and provides strategies that can be used to interact assertively and effectively.

Chapter 7 takes a creative approach to difficulties that often occur at work, and helps us to see them differently, and thus respond to them thoughtfully.

Chapter 8 shows us positive ways to approach busy workplaces, so that they become rewarding, enriching, and stimulating places to work.

Chapter 9 reminds us of important self-caring strategies that replenish and renew us after stressful encounters.

Chapter 10 examines the coping strategies that can be harnessed and used effectively when we face workplace crises.

Chapter 11 discusses nurses who exemplify good leadership to reveal qualities that can be integrated by others.

Chapter 12 brings us back to our initial reflections on resilience for practice in the health professions and offers some concluding thoughts.

As an added resource for nursing instructors, we have produced an online companion to the book. The companion provides instructors with additional activities and questions that can be used to promote reflection, stimulate discussion, and inspire learners to take effective action in their professional lives.

Each of the chapters in the book reveals how nursing is an exciting, a rewarding, and a responsible work. If you are like other nursing students, then you've chosen this career because you sincerely want to care for others. You want to make a difference. However, remember that to be forewarned is to be forearmed. That is, there is more to nursing than caring for others. Nursing is a complex and stressful profession in which you will deal with the best of humanity—and sometimes the worst. You will bear witness to other people's pain and you may even experience vicarious trauma. To emerge positively and grow from all of these challenges, you will need to draw on the special quality of *resilience*. This book shows you how to strengthen your resilience for the exciting journey ahead!

Acknowledgment

We wish to acknowledge and thank Dr. Leigh Findlay for her diligent editorial assistance.

Preparing for Practice: Becoming Resilient

Margaret McAllister and John B. Lowe

Nursing involves complex caring work and the self can flourish in this altruistic experience, but it can also suffer. If you aren't prepared for the emotional and cognitive labour involved with caring, then nursing work can become a burden, leading to stress, burnout, and neglectful care. Let's take a closer look at the causes of workplace stress, and how you can prepare yourself, so that *you* don't wind up as a casualty. We will find that the quality of *resilience* is vitally important.

THE STORY

My name is Josie and I am turning 40 this year. I look back on my life and feel proud of what I've achieved so far. I have finally graduated as a registered nurse (RN), something I've wanted to do for many years.

I had always been a high achiever at school, but I had lots of stress around me. As a child, I read a lot and stayed in my room because my parents had a very volatile marriage. As I got older, I tried to protect my mother from my violent father, which meant I sometimes ended up being beaten myself. I started to blink my eyes a lot, a nervous habit that the teachers picked up, and I developed a social phobia. I would not speak in public places because I was always ridiculed for my poor pronunciation. My father used to criticise me and put me down in front of people. I felt really embarrassed and demoralised.

I finished a nursing course at 19 and then began a Bachelor of Applied Science. I only managed to complete 6 months of this degree because I fell pregnant with my first child. I kept working up until 4 weeks before

I had Daniel. He was the best thing I had ever seen. Beautiful and all mine. I adored him. I stayed with his dad, which wasn't a whole lot of fun and had Sam 2 years later. I went back to work 6 months after having both children, because we needed the money. I broke up with their father while my children were still young. He was becoming like my own father and I didn't want my boys to live like that. I needed to take some time off because I couldn't face work. I felt so worn out and didn't have the energy to help others; so I talked to my nursing supervisor. She had just been through cancer. She listened and helped me solve my problem.

I ended up moving house. The kids started at a new school and fitted in well. I got a job as a wound care nurse in a nursing home and then completed my degree in nursing. I did well and enjoyed it. That is the achievement I'm most proud of. It was something I had waited a long time for. I sometimes still have anxiety attacks in public. I feel them coming on but have learned how to control them now. I started to feel empowered by this. I was finally doing something for myself and doing it well. I became a preceptor at work and started helping others who were being bullied and new staff who needed my support.

Since starting my graduate year, I have had a rather nasty encounter with bullying in the workplace myself. I was shouted at, called names, and belittled in front of everyone. In the past, I would have let it go, but this time I didn't. At first, I cried all night, but then I thought, "No. I won't accept this." The next day, I confronted the person and told her it was unacceptable behaviour, and if it continued, I would be going formal with a complaint. It worked! She has been very quiet since. I am now working in an acute mental health inpatient unit. I love working with the patients. I find it rewarding and challenging. The little things, like being told by the patients that you made them feel important or made time for them, are the things I like. Even on the busiest days, I try to make time to talk with each of my patients and ask them how they are feeling. I try to find out something about their lives, not just their symptoms.

LEARNING FROM THE STORY

The story you have read is true and we sincerely thank the nurse who graciously gave her permission to have it paraphrased here. We think it is apt because there are elements within it to which many readers will relate: particular life experiences that influence the decision to become a nurse; life struggles that continue throughout a career, making us at times vulnerable to stress and burnout; and personal life events that can be used to make your work more meaningful. Nursing, like all other human service work, is at once both taxing and deeply rewarding. This story also touches on the serious reality that nursing can be associated with adversity and trauma, a concept explored in detail in Chapter 10.

STRESS AND THE IMPORTANCE OF RESILIENCE

Expectations of Today's Nurses

Being prepared for the challenges ahead may make all the difference in preventing undue stress and in increasing success. An important element to consider is what employers may expect from you. As a 21st-century nursing graduate, it is likely that your expectations and needs as a worker differ from those of previous generations. Unfortunately, the large bureaucracies characteristic of many health services can be slow to respond to changing needs (Hodges, Keeley, & Grier, 2005). The challenge of thriving in the workplace is explored in detail in Chapter 8.

> Being prepared for the challenges ahead may make all the difference in preventing undue stress and in increasing success.

Holmes (2006) has described several characteristics typical of today's young workers (Table 1.1). Now, if we add to some of the negative characteristics of the typical health bureaucracy (Table 1.2), then we have the perfect recipe for conflict, stress, burnout, and neglectful care (Holmes, 2006). Perhaps this is why some progressive health services are now instituting employee-friendly policies and practices and marketing themselves as great places to work (Figure 1.1).

Sources of Stress

Aside from having to work in a bureaucracy, sources of stress in nursing work are numerous. Rising patient acuity, rapid assessments and

TABLE 1.1   Characteristics of the Y Generation

- Likely to have received a full high school education
- Envision many careers during their lifetime
- Technology rich and multimedia literate
- Time poor
- Impatient
- High expectations of employers:
  - Expect autonomy in the job
  - Less accepting of seniority
  - Expect performance-based remuneration
  - Orientated towards results
- Value work–life balance
- Unlikely to have loyalty to one employer

Source: Adapted from Holmes (2006).

discharges, and increased service use by clients mean that nurses are dealing with sicker people who are likely to have multiple conditions that may complicate both the treatment and the recovery (Gaynor, Gattasch, Yorkston, Stewart, & Turner, 2006). These pressures can lead to work-role overload and burnout.

Therefore, the health service that you join is unlikely to be the comfortable, predictable, friendly place that is depicted in television shows like *Scrubs*. For a start, the people in teams will probably change quite rapidly. Certainly, the client turnaround will be fast. You may be quite regularly rostered to new areas to fill workforce gaps. Hence,

TABLE 1.2   Negative Features of Large Bureaucracies

- Uneven staff skill mix
- Rapid staff turnover and instability
- Work conditions are employer focused
- Economics is the bottom line (consequences include widespread unpaid overtime)
- Disparaging and rigid management
- Controlling (leading to limited worker autonomy)

Source: Adapted from Holmes (2006).

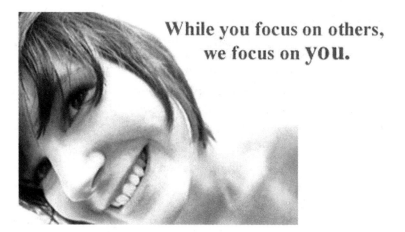

FIGURE 1.1   Advertisement for recruiting nurses.

understanding more about stress, and ways to reduce, manage, or overcome it, will be an important asset to you.

[Understanding more about stress will be an important asset to you.]

The Stress Diathesis Model

The stress diathesis model suggests that accumulation of stress can lead to health breakdown (Figure 1.2). The model also proposes that people must first have a biological, psychological, or sociocultural predisposi-

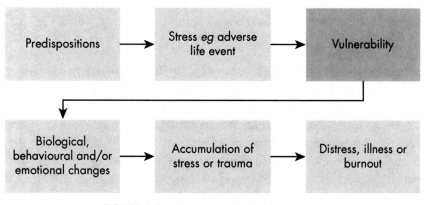

FIGURE 1.2   The stress diathesis model.

tion to such disorders and must then be subjected to an immediate stressor to develop disease or abnormality (Fontaine & Fletcher, 2003).

Now, most people go through life with predispositions to various disorders that are never expressed. What protects them from succumbing to stress or what methods they use to moderate stress are important to understand and underscore the significance of another important concept—*resilience.*

Defining Resilience

The concept of resilience refers to a person's *resistance* to stress. Resilience has been defined in various ways such as an *ability* to rebound from adversity and overcome difficult circumstances in one's life (Marsh, 1996); a *process* of adaptation to adversity (Newman, 2003); and a complex concept that combines individual, family, or organisational *characteristics.*

> Resilience is a process of adapting to adversity that can be developed and learned.

Research Into Resilience

A historical review of the resilience research shows that the concept of resilience has undergone definitional changes, and that various aspects have been subject to research (McAllister & McKinnon, 2009). The conceptual development of resilience dates back to the 1800s, when comment was made on the ability of some people to endure hardship better than others. However, it was not until the 1970s that work on resilience in health and illness began (Luthar, Cicchetti, & Becker, 2000).

Resilient Children
Initially, research was undertaken to explore children of parents diagnosed with schizophrenia (Billings & Moos, 1983), which later became the more inclusive study of children of parents with mental illness (COPMI). These children, dependent on parents for emotional, social, and physical wellbeing, are very vulnerable to parental inconsistency and neglect. When they experience these conditions, they often develop learning difficulties and social and mental health problems (Worland, Weeks, & Janes, 1987).

Further studies involved marginalised children and adolescents who had experienced low socioeconomic circumstances, abuse, parental mental and chronic illness, violent communities, or tragic life incidents (Aronowitz, 2005; Jacelon, 1997). These studies showed that, within communities, young people deal with and overcome adversity better and are able to envision a future for themselves when there is *social connection* with family, peers, and other adults; when there is positive *role modelling* of winners or achievers; when there is unobtrusive *monitoring* of their wellbeing; and when there is *coaching* to help set goals and elevate expectations (Table 1.3).

TABLE 1.3   Risk and Protective Factors in Children

Risk Factors	**Protective Factors**
1. Poor physical health	1. Physical wellbeing, good nutrition, sleep, and exercise
2. Low self-esteem	2. Self-esteem
3. Insecure or unsafe accommodation	3. Secure, appropriate, and safe accommodation
4. Exposure to physical and emotional violence	4. Physical and emotional security
5. Harmful alcohol, tobacco, and other drug use	5. No harmful alcohol, tobacco, and other drug use
6. Feeling disconnected from family, school, and community	6. Positive school climate and achievement; supportive caring parent(s)
7. Lack of meaningful daily activities	7. Meaningful daily activities
8. Poor problem-solving skills	8. Problem-solving skills
9. Lack of control over one's life	9. Sense of control and efficacy
10. Financial hardship	10. Financial security
11. Exposure to environmental stressors (e.g., school bullying)	11. Lack of exposure to environmental stressors
12. Poor social skills	12. Prosocial peers
13. Parental mental illness	13. Optimism
14. Learning difficulties	14. Involvement with significant other person
15. Family divorce or separation	15. Availability of opportunities at critical turning points or major life transitions
16. Poor coping skills	16. Good coping skills

Source: Adapted from Bogenschneider (1996).

Resilient Adults

Resilience research has now extended to adults. For example, research in people with schizophrenia ascertained that those with less severe symptoms were more likely to have positive outcomes in the areas of employment, responsibilities, and social relations, including marriage (Luthar et al., 2000). These insights supported mental health interventions that targeted social and occupational factors, in addition to symptom management. They also prompted thinking on factors to support wellbeing and productivity in other groups. A paradigm shift for health practitioners began. For many, this has meant a reorientation from a concern only for illness to also considering wellbeing.

Aaron Antonovsky (1987) introduced the term *salutogenesis* to describe a focus that supports health and wellbeing rather than focusing on factors that cause disease. The concept has influenced public health (Gregg & O'Hara, 2007), psychology (Suedfeld, 2005), and some areas of nursing (Horsfall & Stuhlmiller, 2000; McAllister & Estefan, 2002). The term salutogenesis comes from the Latin, *salus* meaning health and the Greek, *genesis* meaning origin. Antonovsky studied the influence of various stressors on health and was able to show that relatively unstressed people had much more resistance to illness than those who were more stressed. Antonovsky argued that the experience of wellbeing constitutes a *sense of coherence*. That is, "a pervasive, enduring though dynamic feeling of confidence that one's internal and external environments are predictable and that there is a high probability that things will work out as well as can reasonably be expected" (Antonovsky, 1979, p. 123).

Smith (2002) suggested that a strong sense of coherence assists a person's ability to cope and consists of three factors: meaningfulness—the profound experience that this stressor makes sense in one's life and thus, coping is desirable; manageability—the recognition of the resources required to meet the demands of the situation and a willingness to search out those resources; and comprehensibility—the perception of the world as understandable, meaningful, and orderly and consistent rather than chaotic, random, and unpredictable.

Survivor stories such as the life of Viktor Frankl (1963), Elie Wiesel (1958), and Primo Levi (1979) have inspired work in psychotherapy, philosophy, peace studies, and literature. Frankl, for example, emerged from the Holocaust without the deep emotional injuries found in many survivors of the Nazi death camps. His compassion for his fellow prisoners led him to work at developing ways to help them maintain their will to live.

In fact, this terrible experience ultimately enriched Frankl's life and that of many others. Thus, the long-term consequences of even extreme trauma may include increased personal strength and growth. This phenomenon, now known as *posttraumatic growth*, is a growing area of research within psychology and psychiatry (Linley & Joseph, 2004; Tedeschi & Calhoun, 2004).

Primo Levi wrote an influential book on the ability of the human spirit to rise above suffering. His book has been motivating and inspirational to many who have needed courage to endure. Similarly, Elie Wiesel's famous statement ". . . to remain silent and indifferent is the greatest sin of all . . ." was his life motto as he pursued a lifelong commitment to world peace. In 1986, he was awarded the Nobel Peace Prize.

Another example of thriving through adversity is the story of Lt. Commander Charlie Plumb (1986). Plumb was a navy pilot shot down early in the Vietnam War. He was taken to a prison in Hanoi and kept in a stone cell for 6 years, where he was tortured and deprived. He said of that experience, "It's probably the most valuable six years of my life. Amazing what a little adversity can teach a person. . . . I really felt there was some meaning to that, to my experience itself" (Siebert, 1996, p. 6).

Segal (1986) summarises the significance of this survivor research thus:

> In a remarkable number of cases, those who have suffered and prevail find that after their ordeal they begin to operate at a higher level than ever before. . . . The terrible experiences of our lives, despite the pain they bring, may become our redemption. (p. 130)

In this posttraumatic growth research, much has been learned about the personality and dispositional characteristics of resilient people. Research has explored cancer survivors (Rowland & Baker, 2005), people living with AIDS (Rabkin, Remien, Williams, & Katoff, 1993), people who are ageing (Ryff, Singer, Love, & Essex, 1998), and people who endured the tragedy of the September 11 attacks (Butler et al., 2005).

Coping Skills

Increasing resilience through good coping skills has been researched in recent years, and the concept is more fully explored in Chapters 5 and 9. Smith, Smoll, and Ptacek (1990) found that providing social supports to high school athletes reduced the risk of physical injuries. Greef and Human (2004) found that good coping skills helped children overcome the death of a parent. Walker (2002) found that health care needs may be better met when older adults are able to come to a point of "self-transcendence," wherein they have mastered their stress and accepted or accommodated their stressors.

Personal attributes such as internal locus of control, prosocial behaviour, empathy, positive self-image, optimism, and the ability to organise daily responsibilities enable individuals to build supportive relationships with family members and friends. In stressful periods, resilient individuals will use these attributes to cope with challenges (Friborg, Hjemdal, Rosenvinge, & Martinussen, 2003). Resilient individuals also appear to be more adaptable to change than vulnerable people are. By using protective resources, which are both within and outside the control of the individual, they are able to effectively deal with adversity (Friborg et al., 2003).

Resiliency in adults appears to involve five dimensions. These dimensions are connectedness to one's social environment, connectedness to one's physical environment, connectedness to one's family, connectedness to one's sense of inner wisdom (experiential spirituality), and, also, having a personal psychology with a supportive mindset and a way of living that supports one's values (Denz-Penhey & Murdoch, 2008).

The U.S. resiliency centre, headed by the psychologist Al Siebert (2005), identifies 13 characteristics of resilient people (Table 1.4).

This survivor-focused research is relevant to building resilience in health professionals. Evocative, moving stories from survivors can contribute to others' learning by renewing awareness of the power of the human spirit to endure and overcome and by revealing the value of generative practices such as concern and altruism. Using storytelling may also be a powerful and effective way to "inoculate" students of the health professions against stress and burnout by raising their awareness of resilience strategies and illustrating how to transcend adversity.

Resiliency May Involve Context-Specific Skills

Another view of resilience is the notion that resiliency is contextual and dynamic (Gu & Day, 2007). That is, individuals may not display resilience in all aspects of their lives, and various life transitions may activate different genetically determined biological reactions that require different coping mechanisms, social supports, and spiritual strength.

In addition, some resilience resources may be readily available in some contexts but not in others. For example, social supports may be

TABLE 1.4 Features of Resiliency

1. Playful, childlike curiosity
2. Constantly learn from experience
3. Adapt quickly
4. Solid self-esteem and self-confidence
5. Self-confidence is reputation with oneself
6. Good friendships, loving relationship
7. Express feelings honestly
8. Expect things to work out well
9. Read others with empathy
10. Use intuition, creative hunches
11. Defend self well
12. A talent for serendipity; convert misfortune into good luck and gain
13. Get better and better every decade

Source: Adapted from Siebert (2008).

forthcoming in situations that involve publicly acknowledged crises. However, when a crisis is associated with stigma or shame, then supports may not be accessible, and maintaining resilience may require coping of a different magnitude or quality (Deveson, 2003). From this viewpoint, resilience has an added contextual dimension involving an interaction between the stressor, the context and personal characteristics (Figure 1.3).

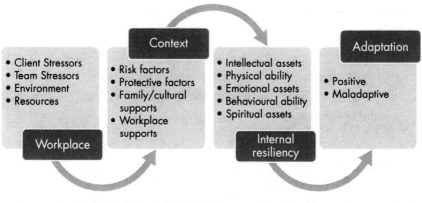

FIGURE 1.3 **A dynamic framework of resilience.**

Resilience Across Cultures and Communities

Resilience has also been viewed as a complex cultural construct that involves a dynamic interaction between individual and family, with maintenance of positive adaptation despite adverse experiences (Luthar et al., 2000). This viewpoint notably includes the concept of the family having group resilience, rather than only individuals demonstrating resilience.

Similar factors have been found to contribute to resilience across cultures. Lothe and Heggen (2003) found resilience in survivors of the Ethiopian famine of 1984–1985 who demonstrated faith, hope, and valued memories of their homeland, and who had a living relative.

Through the study of vulnerable cultures and communities, there is now increased knowledge about community resiliency—that is, the ability of a community to deal with adversity and in so doing, reach a higher level of functioning. Within the U.S. Latino youth population, Clauss-Ehlers and Levi (2002) found particular community resilience factors that protected the young people from violence. These factors included respect for the authority of elders and the value of relationships for their own merit.

Identification with one's cultural group also seems to be important to resilience. Hegney, Eley, Plank, Buikstra, and Parker (2006) have explained the importance of *attachment* to the rural population. Participants in this study identified factors such as attachment to land, family, culture, and community as environmental resources that had assisted them to overcome adversity. The research indicated that participation in community activities promoted the development of social networks that also provided support to less resilient members of the community. This notion of attachment and sense of belonging is likely to be equally relevant to health practitioners.

> Resilient communities transcend adversity because of community members feeling bonded to each other and to the community.

Resilience at Work

This broader view of resilience has also been applied to the work context. Resilience frameworks to assist employees within organisations have been developed (Walsh, 2003), and campaigns aimed at the public have been launched (Newman, 2003). Both aim to boost resilience in people experiencing life stressors. In Australia in 2006, a leading telecommunication company, Telstra, launched a campaign to develop resilience in its employees. The campaign's main approach has been to provide employees with a 56-page glossy document that details strategies individuals can use to relax, to challenge self-defeating thoughts using Cognitive Behavioural Therapy (CBT), and to deal with conflicts. However, as the health promotion discipline has revealed, information on its own does not necessarily lead to change (Nutbeam, 2000). Individuals, groups, and organisations need to be assisted to apply new knowledge.

A concept within the public health discipline that is yet to be linked to workplace resilience, particularly within the health workforce, is the concept of healthy hospitals (Baum, 2002; Noblet, 2003; World Health Organization, 1997). This concept applies the principles of health promotion not to individuals but to the physical and built environments in which people work and live. The assumption is that supportive, preferred working environments for health workers have the capacity to improve overall health and wellbeing (Baum, 2002). How healthy work environments contribute to overall resilience is an area worthy of investigation, especially as health workplaces are becoming busier with the biotechnology boom increasing turnover of clients and adding to client longevity and their use of health services. How the work environments of health workers can be made more worker-friendly in this dynamic context is an important area for research.

Of course, working in health is not a torturous experience, but it can be an ordeal. Thus, it is important to learn from and to relate these insights about resilience to the wellbeing of health professionals. Clinicians' orientations to the nature of their work and how meaningful it is to their lives would seem to be important. If health work is just a job, as it is for some clinicians, then this attitude may be correlated with lower levels of resilience. Experiences that are significant, or even traumatic, such as the first time a clinician faces the untimely death of a client, must be processed and understood. The coping styles and capabilities that clinicians bring to their work, either through upbringing or through education, may well help them face challenges and even grow from them.

> Healthy work environments have the capacity to improve overall health and wellbeing of the workers.

Resilience in the Health Professions

As resilience is considered a personal and cultural strategy for surviving and even transcending adversity, the concept is now used to explore and understand health professionals who survive and thrive in their workplaces. Jackson, Firtko, and Edenborough (2007), in their review of the literature, explain that resilience is a quality necessary to succeed in nursing because the conditions can be so adverse. Moreover, whilst caring is central to nurses' work, many nurses neglect self-care. We see self-care as an important aspect of resilience. We look at self-care more closely in Chapter 9.

Research within health professional groups who experience high exposure to potentially traumatic experiences, such as emergency nurses and ambulance and paramedic personnel, has found that characteristics such as extroversion, openness, agreeableness, conscientiousness, and good coping strategies influence posttraumatic growth (Shakespeare-Finch, Gow, & Smith, 2005).

Jackson et al. (2007) distilled five strategies to develop resilience in nurses:

- Building positive professional relationships through networks and mentoring
- Maintaining positivity through laughter, optimism, and positive emotions
- Developing the emotional insight to understand one's own risk and protective factors
- Achieving life balance and using spirituality to give one's life meaning and coherence
- Becoming more reflective, which helps access emotional strength and assists in meaning making and thus, in transcending the present ordeal.

These strategies are also directly transferable to other health professionals. Jackson et al. (2007) argue for the need to teach and encourage all health professionals to:

- Identify their own risk and protective factors
- Share experiences of both vulnerability and resilience so that others may learn from—and perhaps emulate—the strengths and also avoid the pitfalls
- Acknowledge and praise success in peers' achievements
- *Promote* feelings of pride

All of these actions will help to build resilience.

Resilience Can Be Learned

Various disciplines have now produced convincing evidence that individuals can learn resilience and acquire resilient qualities. The positive psychology movement has been a leader in this research. Seligman's (1998) work on learned optimism, for example, argued that a person's explanatory style shapes the meaning and the effect of adverse experiences. Moreover, one can learn to be optimistic by using focused cognitive behavioural techniques that dispute pessimistic thinking and thus, become more adaptive and resilient. For example, optimists don't give up as easily and don't see an adverse situation as permanent; optimists think that bad things happen sometimes, not all the time; optimists don't always blame themselves when bad things happen—rather they see that the situation or external factors may have been the cause.

Charney (2004) initially studied resilient Vietnam prisoners of war and identified 10 personality traits that were common to resilient people. He went on to establish evidence that CBT can successfully assist in developing many of these traits (Table 1.5).

Relevance of Resilience Research to Nursing

The resilience research presents some important concepts that are readily applicable to nurses. Most of the literature divides resilience into factors that put people at risk or factors that protect them. Protective factors such as positive coping mechanisms and using social supports and personal spirituality, which are known to help children, youth, older people, and those surviving traumatic experiences, are readily applicable to nurses. Moreover, evidence suggests these qualities may be developed through positive learning experiences.

Some of the risk factors that have been identified in groups such as soldiers, prisoners of war, and displaced or traumatised people may also be directly applicable to nurses. However, exploratory and intervention-based research to examine resilience as a tool for dealing with stress in health care workplaces is only just beginning, and there is much more to discover (Gillespie, Chaboyer, Wallis, & Grimbeek, 2007; Jackson et al., 2007).

An aspect of resilience often overlooked, certainly within the context of the health workplace, is the actions that can be taken and the changes implemented to moderate the impact of stress and adversity on workers' lives. That is, everyone should be proactive about resilience in the workplace. Health care work is always going to be busy, unpredictable, and emotionally demanding of clinicians, and so they will need more than

TABLE 1.5   Characteristics of Resilient People That Can Be Learned or Developed

Character	Description and How to Cultivate the Character
Optimism	▦ Strongly related to resilience
	▦ Optimists usually have decreased autonomic arousal, use more adaptive coping strategies, and seek supportive relationships during crises
	▦ Can be learned through Cognitive Behaviour Therapy
Cognitive flexibility	▦ Ability to restructure knowledge in adaptive ways in response to changing demands
	▦ Reduces incidence of posttraumatic stress disorder after combat
	▦ Speeds recovery after loss of a family member or natural disaster
Personal moral compass	▦ Helps people get through adversity
	▦ Many victims of Hurricane Katrina and 9/11 attributed their survival to faith, either through religion or through spirituality
Altruism	▦ Coping with extreme stress is often made easier by helping others
Having a role model who demonstrates resilience	▦ Find a mentor or heroic figure
	▦ Imitation is a powerful mode of learning; heroic figures inspire us to greatness, even though they might not achieve success
Adeptness at facing fears	▦ Recognise that fear is normal and can be used as a guide
	▦ Practise skills needed to get through your fears
Active coping skills	▦ Create positive statements about the self in relation to a threat
	▦ Seek active support from others
Supportive social network	▦ Value seen dramatically after 9/11 and Hurricane Katrina; intense debriefing doesn't seem to help
	▦ Emotional strength comes from close, meaningful relationships
Physical fitness	▦ Exercise is good for physical wellbeing, and also enhances brain health and plasticity
Sense of humour	▦ Narrows gap between doctors and nurses
	▦ Narrows gap between carers and patients, especially children, who often feel helpless and forlorn
	▦ Helps patients cope with their illness

Source: Adapted from Charney (2004).

good defences. They will need to receive support such as mentoring and education. Survivors of adversity show us how this can be done. Surviving for people like Frankl wasn't about being helped; it was about searching for and finding something resourceful and sustaining deep within the self. Then, it was about giving back to others. This *generativity*, demonstrated by altruism, setting a good example, mentoring, leading, coaching, and motivating others, is a practice that could be learned by and strengthened in those entering the health professions. Instead of seeing generativity as the domain of our elders, we need to realise the inherent value in its practice at all ages.

> Nurses should be proactive about resilience in the workplace. Health care work is busy, unpredictable, and emotionally demanding. Nurses need more than good coping mechanisms.

Furthermore, a systems approach to resilience would assist health practitioners to understand that change can be facilitated in the individual professional, the client, and the health environment. To provide healthy hospital environments and reform workplace cultures, however, political skills such as policy formation and lobbying may need to become core skills for health practitioners as the importance of these issues grows.

We need to use our positive experiences to help others. We also need to learn from our negative experiences: be mindful not to perpetuate negative behaviour we might have experienced by inflicting it on others. By respecting ourselves and others, even if this means stepping out of our comfort zone and trying a different approach in challenging situations, we can build our self-esteem. Moreover, with good self-esteem, anything is possible.

CONCLUSION

The way we approach and view an event determines the outcome, rather than the event itself. Resilience is a complex combination of inherited traits, temperament, and learned coping skills, and is an invaluable quality to help you thrive in your chosen career and in life. Predictors of resilience such as cognitive ability, adaptability, positive identity, social support, coping skills, spiritual connection, ability to find meaning in adversity, and generative skills are all qualities that can be learned or strengthened. Hence, *you* can do something about developing your own resilience. As Josie's story suggests, clinicians who show resilience and posttraumatic growth have the potential to be inspiring role models.

We've learned in this chapter that generativity is a concept usually applied to older adults, who gain fulfilment by sharing their stories, wisdom, and experiences, and thus, help the younger generation avoid mistakes. However, generativity should be equally employed by all of us, regardless of age and experience. As future nurses, you can model generativity by sharing your resilience strategies with those who are less experienced. In this way, you will contribute to halting the intergenerational cycle of oppression of which nurses have sometimes been accused (McKenna, Smith, Poole, & Coverdale, 2003).

Tips to Manage Stress

There are many healthy ways to manage and cope with stress.

You can either **change the situation** or **change your reaction**. As everyone has a unique response to stress, there is no "one-size-fits-all" solution to managing it. No single method works for everyone or in every situation, so experiment with different techniques and strategies. Focus on what makes you feel calm and in control.

Dealing With Stressful Situations: The Four A's

Change the situation:

- ✔ **Avoid** the stressor
- ✔ **Alter** the stressor

Change your reaction:

- ✔ **Adapt** to the stressor.
- ✔ **Accept** the stressor.

LEARNING ACTIVITIES

1. Access the resilience inventory at http://www.resiliencescale .com/. Complete the test and then reflect on your strengths and your vulnerabilities. If you feel comfortable doing so, share these insights with your fellow learners in a group discussion.

2. In the story, Josie fits the description of a "wounded healer"—a clinician who has drawn on her own painful experiences to become a more caring professional. *Wounded healer* is a term that has long been applied to many clinicians (Daneault, 2008; O'Hare, 2002). Indeed, Carl Jung (1989) wrote, "The doctor [*sic*] is effective only when he himself is affected. . . . Only the wounded physician heals. But when the doctor wears his personality like a coat of armour, he has no effect" (p. 134). What do you think he meant by this statement? What can you learn from it about your own life experiences?

3. Access at least one article on the concept of the wounded healer. Use the discussion of this concept to analyse key points within Josie's story and the chapter.

REFERENCES

Antonovsky, A. (1979). *Health, stress, and coping.* San Francisco, CA: Jossey-Bass.

Antonovsky, A. (1987). *Unraveling the mystery of health: How people manage stress and stay well.* San Francisco, CA: Jossey-Bass.

Aronowitz, T. (2005). The role of "envisioning the future" in the development of resilience among at-risk youth. *Public Health Nursing, 22*(3), 200–208.

Baum, F. (2002). *The new public health: An Australian perspective.* South Melbourne, Australia: Oxford University Press.

Billings, A., & Moos, R. (1983). Comparisons of children of depressed and non-depressed parents: A social-environmental perspective. *Journal of Abnormal Child Psychology, 11*(4), 463–486.

Bogenschneider, K. (1996). An ecological risk/protective theory for building prevention programs, policies, and community capacity to support youth. *Family Relations, 45*(2), 127–138.

Butler, L., Blasey, C., Garlan, R., McCaslin, S., Azarow, J., Chen, X., . . . Spiegel, D. (2005). Posttraumatic growth following the terrorist attacks of September 11, 2001: Cognitive, coping, and trauma symptom predictors in an internet convenience sample. *Traumatology, 11*(4), 247-267.

Charney, D. S. (2004). Psychobiological mechanisms of resilience and vulnerability: Implications for successful adaptation to extreme stress. *American Journal of Psychiatry, 161*(2), 195-216.

Clauss-Ehlers, C., & Levi, L. (2002). Violence and community, terms in conflict: An ecological approach to resilience. *Journal of Social Distress and the Homeless, 11*(4), 265-278.

Daneault, S. (2008). The wounded healer. Can this idea be of use to family physicians? *Canadian Family Physician, 54*(9), 1218-1219.

Denz-Penhey, H., & Murdoch, C. (2008). Personal resiliency: Serious diagnosis and prognosis with unexpected quality outcomes. *Qualitative Health Research, 18*(3), 391-404.

Deveson, A. (2003). *Resilience.* Sydney, Australia: Penguin.

Fontaine, K., & Fletcher, S. (2003). *Mental health nursing* (5th ed.). Upper Saddle River, NJ: Pearson.

Frankl, V. (1963). *Man's search for meaning.* New York, NY: Washington Square Press.

Friborg, O., Hjemdal, O., Rosenvinge, J., & Martinussen, M. (2003). A new rating scale for adult resilience: What are the central protective resources behind healthy adjustment? *International Journal of Methods in Psychiatric Research, 12*(2), 65-77.

Gaynor, L., Gattasch, T., Yorkston, E., Stewart, S., & Turner, C. (2006). Where do all the undergraduate and new graduate nurses go and why? A search for empirical research evidence. *Australian Journal of Advanced Nursing, 24*(2), 26-32.

Gillespie, B., Chaboyer, W., Wallis, M., & Grimbeek, P. (2007). Resilience in the operating room: Developing and testing of a resilience model. *Journal of Advanced Nursing, 59*(4), 427-438.

Greef, A., & Human, B. (2004). Resilience in families in which a parent has died. *American Journal of Family Therapy, 32*(1), 27-42.

Gregg, J., & O'Hara, L. (2007). Values and principles evident in current health promotion practice. *Health Promotion Journal of Australia, 18*(1), 7-11.

Gu, Q., & Day, C. (2007). Teachers' resilience: A necessary condition for effectiveness. *Teaching and Teacher Education, 23*(8), 1302-1316.

Hegney, D., Eley, R., Plank, A., Buikstra, E., & Parker, V. (2006). Workforce issues in nursing in Queensland: 2001 and 2004. *Journal of Clinical Nursing, 15*(12), 1521-1530.

Hodges, H. F., Keeley, A. C., & Grier, E. C. (2005). Professional resilience, practice longevity, and Parse's theory for baccalaureate education. *Journal of Nursing Education, 44*(12), 548-554.

Holmes, C. (2006). The slow death of psychiatric nursing: What next? *Journal of Psychiatric and Mental Health Nursing, 13*(4), 401–415.

Horsfall, J., & Stuhlmiller, C. (2000). Saluting health: The imperative of nursing and mental health nursing. In J. Horsfall & C. Stuhlmiller (Eds.), *Interpersonal nursing for mental health* (pp. 97–124). New York, NY: Springer Publishing Company Inc.

Jacelon, C. (1997). The trait and process of resilience. *Journal of Advanced Nursing, 25*(1), 123–129.

Jackson, D., Firtko, A., & Edenborough, M. (2007). Personal resilience as a strategy for surviving and thriving in the face of workplace adversity: A literature review. *Journal of Advanced Nursing, 60*(1), 1–9.

Jung, C. (1989). *Memories, dreams, reflections.* New York, NY: Vintage Books.

Levi, P. (1979). *If this is a man.* London, England: Penguin.

Linley, P. A., & Joseph, S. (2004). Positive change following trauma and adversity: A review. *Journal of Traumatic Stress, 17*(1), 11–21.

Lothe, E., & Heggen, K. (2003). A study of resilience in young Ethiopian famine survivors. *Journal of Transcultural Nursing, 14*(4), 313–320.

Luthar, S., Cicchetti, D., & Becker, B. (2000). The construct of resilience: A critical evaluation and guidelines for future work. *Child Development, 27*(3), 543–562.

Marsh, D. T. (1996). Marilyn . . . and other offspring. *Journal of the California Alliance for the Mentally Ill, 7*(3), 4–6.

McAllister, M., & Estefan, A. (2002). Principles and strategies for teaching therapeutic responses to self-harm. *Journal of Psychiatric and Mental Health Nursing, 9*(5), 573–583.

McAllister, M., & McKinnon, J. (2009). The importance of teaching and learning resilience in the health disciplines: A critical review of the literature. *Nurse Education Today, 29,* 371–379.

McKenna, B., Smith, N., Poole, S., & Coverdale, J. (2003). Horizontal violence: Experiences of registered nurses in their first year of practice. *Journal of Advanced Nursing, 42*(1), 90–96.

Newman, R. (2003). Providing direction on the road to resilience. *Behavioral Health Management, 23*(4), 42–43.

Noblet, A. (2003). Building health promoting work settings: Identifying the relationship between work characteristics and occupational stress in Australia. *Health Promotion International, 18*(4), 351–359.

Nutbeam, D. (2000). Health literacy as a public health goal: A challenge for contemporary health education and communication strategies into the 21st century. *Health Promotion International, 15*(3), 259–267.

O'Hare, M. (2002). *The nurse as wounded healer: From trauma to transcendence.* New York, NY: New York University.

Plumb, C. (1986). *I'm not a hero.* P.O. Box 223, Kansas City.

Rabkin, J., Remien, R., Williams, J., & Katoff, L. (1993). Resilience in adversity among long-term survivors of AIDS. *Hospital and Community Psychiatry*, *44*(2), 162–167.

Rowland, J., & Baker, F. (2005). Resilience of cancer survivors across the lifespan. *Cancer*, *101*(11 Suppl.), 2543–2548.

Ryff, R., Singer, B., Love, G., & Essex, M. (1998). Resilience in adult and later life. In J. Lomranz (Ed.), *Handbook of aging and mental health: An integrative approach* (pp. 69–96). New York, NY: Plenum Press.

Segal, J. (1986). *Winning life's toughest battles* (p. 130). New York, NY: McGraw-Hill.

Seligman, M. (1998). *Learned optimism*. New York, NY: Random House.

Shakespeare-Finch, J., Gow, K., & Smith, S. (2005). Personality, coping and post-traumatic growth in emergency ambulance personnel. *Traumatology*, *11*(4), 325–334.

Siebert, A. (1996). *The survivor personality*. Berkley, CA: Perigee Books.

Siebert, A. (2005). *The resiliency advantage*. Portland, OR: Practical Psychology Press, Inc.

Smith, D. (2002). Functional salutogenic mechanisms of the brain. *Perspectives in Biology and Medicine*, *45*(3), 319–328.

Smith, R., Smoll, F., & Ptacek, J. (1990). Conjunctive moderator variables in vulnerability and resiliency research: Life stress, social support and coping skills, and adolescent sport injuries. *Journal of Personality and Social Psychology*, *58*, 360–369.

Suedfeld, P. (2005). Invulnerability, coping, salutogenesis, integration: Four phases of space psychology. *Aviation Space Environmental Medicine*, *76*(Suppl. 6), B61–B66.

Tedeschi, R.G., & Calhoun, L.G. (2004). Posttraumatic growth: Conceptual foundations and empirical evidence. *Psychological Inquiry*, *15*(1), 1–18.

Walker, C. (2002). Transformative aging: How mature adults respond to growing older. *Journal of Theory Construction and Testing*, *6*(2), 109–116.

Walsh, F. (2003). Family resilience: A framework for clinical practice. *Family Process*, *42*(1), 1–18.

Wiesel, E. (1958). *Night*. New York, NY: Hill & Wang.

Worland, J., Weeks, D. G., & Janes, C. L. (1987). Predicting mental health in children at risk. In E. J. Anthony & B. J. Cohler (Eds.), *The invulnerable child* (pp. 185–210). New York, NY: Guilford Press.

World Health Organization. (1997). *The Vienna recommendations on health promoting hospitals*. Retrieved March 12, 2010, from http://www.hphconferences.org/archive/vienna07/htm/hph.htm

(2) Nurses Who Made a Difference

Margaret McAllister and
John B. Lowe

INTRODUCTION

Leadership, according to De Pree (2004), is the art of motivating a group of people to act toward achieving a common goal. Even though this is not a history book, what better way to illustrate the leadership skills we are talking about than to show you the evidence from stories of nursing's past? Storytelling is a powerful way to communicate insights. Good stories are usually far more memorable than disembodied lists or protocols. Further, the meanings that can be made from stories are not fixed or static. The lessons that you or others find important within this chapter might vary considerably from the lessons we uncovered because the reading of a story is an active meaning-making process.

There are many inspirational people in nursing's past: some of them familiar to nurses all over the world, others well known only to some. Nightingale and Seacole, both legendary figures in nursing's history, were contemporaries who lived their working lives in Europe during the Victorian era. Whilst their paths crossed on several occasions, they were never friends and their lives took very different courses.

Nightingale (1820–1910) was christened Florence after the Italian town in which she was born (Figure 2.1). Growing up in England, she was homeschooled by her father. Her family was wealthy, upper class, and socially connected. Her grandfather was the abolitionist, William Smith. At an early age, Florence said that she had a Christian calling to become a nurse, much to the outrage of her parents. Nurses at that time

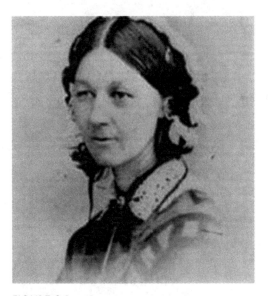

FIGURE 2.1   Florence Nightingale.
Source: Retrieved from www.military
images.net

were not respected, and their role was more that of a cleaner than one caring for patients. Certainly, nursing at the time was not a career for respectable women. However, with Florence's devotion, commitment, and leadership, the profession advanced significantly.

During the Crimean War, in which she volunteered to work whilst in her early 30s, Florence earned the moniker "The Lady with the Lamp" for her reputation for making her rounds of wounded soldiers at night, alone, with only a lamp to light the darkness. Although this war between European nations lasted only for 3 years, it is remembered for revealing military incompetence and for prompting technological reforms such as the telegraph and the tactical use of railways. Being able to immediately send messages home from the war heralded the important role of war correspondents. These reporters exposed the scandalous treatment of wounded soldiers, and showcased the major health reforms performed by the women who served as army nurses. The correspondents also revealed that many of the diseases from which the soldiers were dying were in fact contracted within hospitals because of the unsanitary conditions. Contaminated water, overcrowding, rat infestations, and lack of hand washing were major problems presented in the concepts of germ theory; contagion and hygiene were virtually unknown at this time. Instead, the miasma theory (Corbin, 1996) held sway. This theory blamed diseases such as cholera and the Black Death on miasmas, or "bad air," rather than infections passed by human-to-human contact. Nightingale also believed in the miasma theory, which is why she insisted on fresh air and strict cleanliness. Fortunately, these practices did result in better health outcomes, not by ridding the environment of poisonous air, but rather because they reduced cross-infection. At this time, nurses had no real structure to their work. With Nightingale's insistence and vision, they were given uniforms and training, and were instructed to perform strict routines to improve the sanitation and the personal care of patients. Most of her efforts were not supported by mainstream medicine. She would have faced resistance and criticism for making change, and she would have needed strong resiliency skills to survive.

> Leadership is the art of motivating a group of people to act toward achieving a common goal, and a key resiliency skill—something Florence Nightingale embodied.

Mary Seacole (1805–1881), was born in Kingston, Jamaica (Figure 2.2). Her father was Scottish and her mother was Jamaican and, whilst the family was not wealthy, they also enjoyed a high social status. Mary learned about herbal remedies and folk medicine from her mother who ran a boarding house for disabled soldiers. She overcame several traumas whilst young: In the 1830s, she married a merchant, but he was sickly and his business did not prosper; in the 1840s, her family's boarding house burned down; then, her mother died, followed by her husband. For a short while, Mary took to her bed in grief, but soon composed herself, taking over her mother's business and expanding her nursing skills by travelling through the British colonies. Here she encountered and managed several epidemics of cholera and yellow fever.

Learning about the Crimean war and yearning for more adventure and an opportunity to enjoy "pomp, pride, and circumstance of glorious war" (Seacole & Salih, 1857/2005), Mary travelled to Britain to volunteer as an army nurse. However, perhaps because of prejudice, she was refused. When Nightingale successfully convinced the army to allow a group of female nurses to go to the Crimea, Mary was not amongst those selected. Perhaps, Nightingale did not consider Mary's colour, lack of class, and

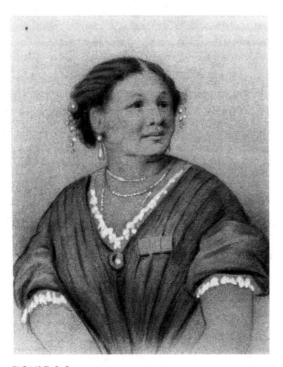

FIGURE 2.2   Mary Seacole. *Source:* Retrieved
from www.militaryimages.net

education fitting. However, not to be deterred, Seacole borrowed money
to travel to the war zone and there she set up a private hotel for British
soldiers. Nightingale reportedly disapproved of Seacole's establishment
because such places allowed gambling, drinking, and prostitution. Whilst
Nightingale and the other nurses stayed within the confines of the army
hospital, Seacole frequently ventured out onto the battlefield, selling
goods and caring for wounded soldiers from both sides.

Thanks to the stories generated by war correspondents and communicated by telegraph, both women became famous, acclaimed as hero-
ines for their bravery and selflessness during the war. Florence returned
to wealth, family, and status, which gave her influence with royalty and
government. This influence enabled her to establish the Nightingale
Training School at St Thomas' Hospital, and to be appointed to commis-
sions to reform health and social services. Mary, however, by the end of
the war was almost destitute, and was only saved from adversity by
friends and benefactors.

Whilst these women lived very different lives, both maintained a lifelong interest in public health. Mary wrote a best seller, the colourfully entitled book, *Wonderful Adventures of Mrs. Seacole in Many Lands* (1857). Florence also wrote several books and was a prolific letter writer, particularly to newspapers. The text *Notes on Nursing* (Nightingale, 1860/2009) became a primer for students of nursing, and was also a best seller. Whilst Florence is known across the world as the founder of modern nursing, Mary struggled against poverty and racism, and after her death she was forgotten for almost a century.

Today, however, Nightingale and Seacole have been immortalised: schools of nursing, scholarships, bursaries, and statues commemorate them both. The Florence Nightingale Museum sits on the grounds of the old St Thomas' Hospital in London. Thousands of nurses remember making the Nightingale pledge after they were given their nursing badge on graduation. The pledge was developed in the United States by Lystra Gretter (1893). It reads:

> I solemnly pledge myself before God and in the presence of this assembly, to pass my life in purity and to practice my profession faithfully. I will abstain from whatever is deleterious and mischievous, and will not take or knowingly administer any harmful drug. I will do all in my power to maintain and elevate the standard of my profession, and will hold in confidence all personal matters committed to my keeping and all family affairs coming to my knowledge in the practice of my calling. With loyalty will I endeavour to aid the physician in his work, and devote myself to the welfare of those committed to my care. (para. 1)

Affirmations are the modern equivalent of the Nightingale pledge. They identify direction that you aim to follow and foster self-belief—a key resiliency skill.

So, what can we learn from Nightingale and Seacole? Kouzes and Posner (1995) list five fundamental practices of exemplary leaders:

- Challenging the process
- Inspiring a shared vision
- Enabling others to act
- Modelling the way
- Encouraging the heart

Both women's lives encapsulate each of these behaviours. A single word describes the quality that helped them endure hostility, doubt, ignorance, and prejudice—strength.

STRENGTH IN NURSING

Being strong as a nurse has many meanings on which reflection is helpful. In some contexts, the strong nurse is someone who has physical power: being on your feet all day, and moving immobilised or dependent patients can be very hard work. Having a strong stomach can also come in handy! One can only imagine the stench, muck, and horror that Nightingale and Seacole must have encountered in their work during the war.

These women also cultivated strength in others; many soldiers recounted stories of how the women encouraged them, in different ways, to stay strong, to stay alive. One story tells that soldiers would blow kisses at Nightingale's shadow as she made her nightly rounds. In contrast, Seacole and her colleagues would host horse-racing carnivals and feasts during rest days to bolster the soldiers' spirits.

Despite many obstacles, including a conservative and sexist society, both women continued to make social reforms. They possessed strength of character, vision, and commitment that is inspiring. Nightingale, especially, had strong social connections that allowed her to make significant changes. She unashamedly capitalised on her networks to achieve the infrastructure necessary to set up training schools for nurses and doctors.

> Nightingale and Seacole embodied a key resiliency quality—strength—which was manifest in different ways.

CONCLUSION

Leadership, a crucial ingredient of resilience, is the recurring theme in this chapter. We have discussed the importance of actions *as well as* words for being an effective influential person. Two historical nursing figures have been mentioned—Nightingale and Seacole—who each, in different ways, showed leadership. We have proposed that one does not have to directly experience adversity to become strong and to be prepared. We hope these stories about the way these women lived their lives may inspire and empower your future nursing practice.

LEARNING ACTIVITIES

1. Visit the Florence Nightingale Museum on the web, located at http://www.florence-nightingale.co.uk/index.php, to learn more about this inspirational leader and her contribution to the nursing profession.

2. Recall and then record a story of a good leader you have known. To complete this activity, use some or all of the following descriptors to help you richly describe your experience:

   a. What characterized the situation?

   b. Who was involved?

   c. Where and when did it take place?

   d. Who initiated the changes?

   e. What was the result?

   f. What lessons did you learn about leadership from this experience?

3. For discussion: Think about the leadership qualities you might possess.

   a. Are there some similarities you share with the nursing leaders?

   b. Can you think of times when you conducted yourself in a manner similar to the way these leaders conducted themselves?

REFERENCES

Corbin, A. (1996). *The foul & the fragrant: Odour & the social imagination.* London, England: Macmillan and Co. Ltd.

De Pree, M. (2004). *Leadership is an art.* New York, NY: Random House.

Gretter, L. (1893). The Nightingale pledge. *A Tribute to Florence Nightingale.* Retrieved from http://www.countryjoe.com/nightingale/pledge.htm

Kouzes, J., & Posner, B. (1995). *The leadership challenge.* San Francisco, CA: Jossey-Bass.

Nightingale, F. (1860/2009). *Notes on nursing: What it is and what it is not.* London, England: Barnes & Noble Publishing.

Seacole, M., & Salih, S. (Eds.). (1857/2005). *Wonderful adventures of Mrs. Seacole in many lands.* London, England: Penguin Classics.

(3) Moral and Ethical Practice

Andrew Estefan

INTRODUCTION

Health care today demands nurses to be technically proficient, competent practitioners who are attuned to the health and social care needs of patients. As we, nurses, seek to meet patients' needs, we are required to practise ethically, and the professional codes of conduct use ethical guidelines to help us formulate appropriate nursing care. Ethical practice is fundamental to safeguarding patients' wellbeing and promotes a therapeutic, trusting relationship between nurses and patients. But what does this really mean? What does an ethical nurse look like, and what do ethical nurses do that makes them so ethical? How do nurses know the *right* thing to do?

This chapter explores nursing ethics and the challenges of nursing ethically. This exploration begins with a story of caring for Jenny, a young woman with anorexia. The story shows how ethical nursing practice can be framed in different ways. Being able to apply ethical reasoning in various patient care situations is one way that nurses can consider options for care and improve the quality of the nurse–patient encounter. At the end of the chapter, you will be presented with some questions and learning activities to help you to think about what ethical practice means to you and how you want to incorporate ethics into your frameworks for practice.

THE STORY

Jenny's Shoes

One morning shift many years ago, I was told I was being assigned as the primary nurse for Jenny, a young woman with anorexia. She had had several previous admissions and had developed a good strong reputation for being a "problem" patient. I was new to the ward and the senior staff felt that a new face might have a different approach, something new to offer. I was briefed about Jenny's past admissions and was warned that she self-injured and could be angry and aggressive, and that she was a "runner." The best advice my colleagues could give me was to see what shoes Jenny was wearing that day—if she had her trainers on, I should expect a less than easy shift! Jenny was admitted 2 days later, and for some weeks, I kept my eye on her choice of footwear.

Jenny would not eat, preferred not to talk about her anorexia, and continued to attempt self-injury. She warned me that she could not be trusted to comply with any of the ward routines or rules, and that her willingness to stay was only influenced by her worry for her mother, who was not coping well with Jenny's deteriorating health. As the new nurse with a different approach, I proposed some strategies for helping Jenny adapt to the environment and trust me enough to start to talk about what was important to her. My approach was met with scepticism and criticism from some of the staff.

> Jenny did not fit into the category of a "good" patient. A good patient is someone who complies with a care plan, who does not actively resist treatment, and who is willing to self-explore. Like many other patients who do not or cannot meet these ideals, Jenny became a "problem" patient.
>
> Rather than consign Jenny to an unhelpful category—problem patient—it may be more helpful to understand her as someone having some difficulty in developing relationships and committing to positive change. Modelling communication, acceptance, and commitment to Jenny is one way a nurse can be helpful here.

My experience of trying to find an effective way to care for Jenny that did not marginalise her experiences was difficult for me. I remember feeling frustrated by being criticised and scrutinised for wanting to find an effective way to work therapeutically with her. This sense of upset that I experienced has a name, and it is a topic that is becoming more prominent in the nursing literature. *Moral distress* is a term that resonates with nurses who find themselves involved in the increasingly complex technical and social environments in which caring occurs today. At present, nursing demands technical skill, proficiency, and emotional literacy, so nursing can be stressful in various ways. Moral distress is what occurs when nurses believe they know the right course of action for a patient, but are unable to follow it (Austin, Kelecevic, Goble, & Mekechuk, 2009; Jameton, 1984). Moral distress is characterised by uncertainty, a sense of powerlessness, anxiety, and frustration of being unable to find a way out of the problem situation (Jameton, 1984). In order for us nurses to work in stressful situations and still feel able to care (and keep caring), we need to find ways to manage troubles like moral distress. Before we can start to think about ways to solve the moral and ethical problems of the practice, such as how to care effectively and accountably for people in distress, we first need to review some of the ethical theories and principles that influence nursing practice.

ETHICAL PRINCIPLES FOR PRACTICE

Ethics is a branch of philosophy that seeks to explore questions about what is right and wrong, as well as what people should or should not do (Oberle & Raffin-Bouchal, 2009). Applying ethical principles to practice problems is one way to critically examine care and to fulfill the obligations and requirements of our profession that safeguard patients. Ethical theories help nursing students understand the *rights* and *wrongs* of caring. These rules are reassuring because, if properly applied, ethical reasoning helps us to determine defensible actions when caring for others. These rights and wrongs can also create difficulties, however, when the practice situation just does not seem to "fit" with certain ethical principles or prevailing practices.

Broadly speaking, ethical theories can be descriptive, prescriptive, or applied. *Descriptive* theories tell us what is happening, *prescriptive* theories tell us what we ought to do, and *applied* theories address both of these aspects, usually in a specific context such as nursing. In practice, ethical theories translate into obligations to behave in a certain way. Nurses are required to perform their duty, and ethics provides a framework within which we can understand the nurses' duties. The ethics of duty is also referred to as *deontology*. Deontological theory foregrounds nurses' *obligations* to safeguard patients' wellbeing. For example, the practice of monitoring fluid intake and output is a practice that observes, measures, and reports, but it also helps to safeguard the patient from harm, arguably one objective of good nursing care. To not record fluid intake and output represents a failure on the part of the nurse to perform his or her duty.

Deontology, or the ethics of duty, plays an important part in nursing practice. One central component of deontological theory is the notion of reasonableness. That is to say, *reasonable* people make ethical decisions and act upon them (Kant, 1949; 1788/2002). While this is a simplification of fairly complex ethical theory, it highlights the idea that there has to be a reference point for, or a way to understand what is considered reasonable nursing behaviour in different clinical contexts. For nurses, there are multiple reference points regarding reasonable (and thus, appropriate and ethical) conduct. For example, education, hospital policy, colleague and interprofessional agreement, and, of course, research that seeks to explore the most efficient and useful ways to care for patients are all points of reference for nurses.

> What is appropriate and ethical conduct at one point in time may differ widely at another point. Consider the nurses who participated in the eugenics experiments and involuntary euthanasia of disabled children in Germany, in the early 20th century (see Benedict & Kuhla, 1999).

Another group of ethical theories that organises health care practices are the consequentialist theories. *Consequentialism*, briefly summarised, is about outcomes. Whereas deontological theory calls attention to the right or wrong of a nursing action in terms of duty, consequentialist ethics ties the nursing action to its outcome, result, or effect asking, "Does the outcome justify the action?" Consequentialist ethics seeks a good outcome. *Utilitarianism*, a form of consequentialist ethics, applies the principle of doing the greatest *good* for the greatest number. Although in health care, we might interpret "good" as being the recovery or reduction of pain, the good that is referred to in foundational utilitarian theory is *happiness* or *pleasure*.

Happiness and pleasure are physical and psychosocial phenomena amenable to nursing intervention; for example, implementing nursing measures to reduce pain and discomfort. Importantly, promoting happiness and pleasure for patients goes beyond physical interventions to attending closely to patients' psychosocial dimensions. But how does a busy and sometimes underresourced nurse work adaptively with patients in this way? After all, many health care settings are extremely busy and demanding contexts for nurses. It may be that nurses need to stop and ask *who are we* and *how are we* with our patients.

Virtue ethics emphasises precisely this aspect of practice. Virtue ethics begins with the assumption that virtuous or good people make ethical decisions. Virtue ethics is about character, but it is also about what drives or motivates us to care (Greenfield & Banja, 2009). Nelson and Gordon (2006) suggested that nurses have a very strong virtue script, which is reinforced by society. That is to say, nurses are seen as possessing certain characteristics that are important in caring for others. The difficulty this creates for nurses is that these characteristics are viewed as being at odds with other virtues such as being assertive, knowledgeable, independent, and proficient.

As we nurses grapple with questions about what to *do* to care for patients while demonstrating our expertise and value, virtue ethics also calls upon us to consider the sort of nurses we want to be. Virtue ethics helps us to focus on what we do and how we cultivate and enact practice values and behaviours that match with and join together our sense of *self as person* and *self as nurse*. In essence, this involves writing a new virtue script: one that claims the ability and capacity to care, and blends this with our personal or self-knowledge and our knowledge and expertise gained from education.

REPOSITIONING ETHICS AND MORALITY IN NURSING

Being a nurse in a caring relationship with someone else creates a new lens through which we can think about ethical practice. Oberle & Raffin-Bouchal (2009) suggest that for nurses, ". . . practice is the moral foundation for nursing ethics" (p. 43). That is to say, that understanding what is ethical or good in nursing is reached through the "doing" of nursing a patient. In addition, nursing occurs in the context of a therapeutic relationship, rather than in the context of a policy or care pathway. Thinking about practice as a relationship in this way causes us to pause and reflect on who we are in that relationship.

Being aware of who we are and what brought us to our privileged position of caring for people when they are vulnerable is more than wasteful self-absorption. Instead, it creates a purposeful opportunity for us to reposition ourselves in the caring transaction and to find ways to become effective agents of health promotion, illness remediation, and change. Sometimes, it can be hard to care for patients because of their particular needs, or because of environmental or institutional constraints. At these times, the knowledge of who we are and what we want to be as nurses provides a bridge over which we can walk to reach the patient on the other side. I would suggest this approach leads to a *meeting place* between people, and, in this meeting place, we create an opportunity to care. Approaching patients in this manner promotes ethical and empathetic caring (Slote, 2007) because actions and interactions in this context are guided by the relationship, as well as some of the other principles of good nursing.

ETHICAL NURSING PRACTICE AS A RELATIONAL ENDEAVOUR

As we practice nursing in environments in which processes, algorithms, and care pathways predominate, we are granted the responsibility and the privilege to meet people at their most vulnerable. Completing tick boxes on care pathways is not enough to help nurses practice ethically as moral agents in relationships, however brief, with other people. Although the notion of virtue is important for nurses to understand who we want to be as professionals, we need to briefly consider another type of ethics. *Relational ethics* helps us sustain our sense of movement towards strategies for ethical practice when we feel that we cannot care for patients as we would want.

> Knowledge of who we are, where we came from, and who we want to be provides a bridge over which we can walk to reach the patient on the other side.

Relational ethics has its roots in feminist theory. Feminist ethicists are cautious of ethical positions that ignore women's experiences and ways of knowing. For example, historically, the female virtues of caring and nurturing were considered less important than male virtues like courage. Gilligan (1982) argued that women make ethical decisions based not on principles, but on how those decisions materially and emotionally affect others. For us as nurses, this is not a debate about the differences between men and women. Instead, it emphasises the alternatives for ethical reasoning in nursing practice. With an eye on how the experience of health care can materially and emotionally affect others, nurses can be attuned to issues and difficulties that may arise, while being grounded in a relationship that works effectively on patients' health care needs. Relational ethics is also useful because our connection with the patient helps us to acknowledge and understand that some problems (like toenails and trainers) cannot be solved. Instead, practicing in a relational way means that nurses are in touch with patients. In this context, nurses and patients can adopt a future orientation and work together to discover what needs to be done and what can be done towards recovery or adaptation (Nelson, 2000).

THE ETHICS OF ADOPTING A SOLUTION FOCUS

Taking a solution focus is one strategy that situates nursing practice in a relational ethical framework. Solution-focused nursing views the experience of illness or disorder as a transition that is amenable to nursing intervention (McAllister, 2007). Using solution-focused lens to guide ethical practice—the reason why the patient needs nursing care—becomes the link between who the patient was before illness and who he or she will become. A solution focus uses the shared experience between nurse and patient to create *movement* at this juncture, where there might otherwise be standstill or stagnation from focusing on an insoluble problem.

> A solution-focused ethics of care in nursing focuses on the future for the patient and the role that nursing care can play in facilitating movement towards that future.

Nursing, in a solution-focused way, involves asking questions, delving deeper into the relationship between nurse and patient, and activating mutual resources to effect awareness and change. Perhaps this sounds a little vague, but think about how the very concrete, knowable features of practice like policies and procedures tend not to provide nurses with answers about how to resolve moral distress. Venturing into the less tangible realms of the relationship between nurse and patient holds promise for discovering ways to resolve ethical conflicts and dilemmas. We might not be able to solve a difficult or intractable problem, but we can continue to work towards a better future or outcome for the patient. Viewed in this way, solution-focused strategies are far from impractical. In fact, solution-focused nursing, as part of a relational ethical approach to care, is strongly grounded in context and practice (Gilligan, 1982; McAllister, 2007; Noddings, 2003). Precisely because it is a practical approach, solution-focused nursing leads us to think about our practice differently, to create options for caring—and this is a very good thing.

To illustrate my point, think back to the story of Jenny. Although I couldn't alter what she could not do, together, we had to think about ways to create movement in our therapeutic relationship. When I reflected in supervision about my work with her, I noticed that we shared a keen interest in stories. Jenny told lots of stories; admittedly, most of them were to avoid having to talk about her anorexia. As I thought more about how I wanted to approach my one-on-one time with Jenny, I started to think about how, as a young man, I used to spend a lot of time with my grandmother. During this time, we used to play cards and I would help her with things that she could no longer do for herself. My grandmother was an excellent "autobiographer" and storyteller. I loved listening to her, and as I recollected the experience of listening to her, I realised that the stories my grandmother used to tell were something that united us and made our time together rewarding and rich. So I resolved to try and use stories to create some movement in my therapeutic relationship with Jenny.

At first, Jenny used words to paint a picture of self-hatred, self-destruction, and hopelessness. She shared her stories; I listened and shared my thoughts and impressions and, when it seemed appropriate, I shared some of my own experiences. After some time, she started to talk about herself differently. As she relaxed into talking about her life, she focused more on how her dream was to one day work with animals. It was here that she felt she could make a difference in the world, and the thought of it made her smile. This dream became the starting point for several interactions that examined where she was in her life now, how to get to where she wanted to be, and how to make that manageable. Anorexia had been the stumbling block in our caring work together. Anorexia continued to be present, like the proverbial elephant in the room. However, once it was no longer at the centre of our relationship, Jenny connected with a sense of possibility for the future. As she connected with a different sense of a future self, she began to think about challenging her ingrained anorectic behaviours.

Perhaps then, being an ethical practitioner of nursing involves bringing our humanity and our experiences to the clinical encounter. Had I not allowed my history with my grandmother to form a lens over my understanding of how I cared for Jenny, I might not have used relational ethics. I may, instead, have continued to work in ways that contained her anorectic behaviours. And the likelihood of a therapeutic relationship that enriched both of us and created possibilities for her beyond those she had previously imagined may have been much reduced.

Relational ethics, however, does not mean that we construct a relationship to meet our own emotional needs. Therapeutic relationships are meant to be therapeutic relationships for our patients. Our own experiences are not uncritically laid bare—this is not the purpose of ethical caring. Ethical caring makes therapeutic use of ourselves, and so our experiences become the lens through which we look as we seek to find ways to work well with patients.

THE OPPORTUNITY TO MAKE A DIFFERENCE

Although a solution-focused, relational approach to nursing is a helpful way to work with patients, it is also about finding ways for us, as nurses, to be good to ourselves. When things in practice do not go the way we expect, or would like, this different understanding of the nurse–patient relationship helps us to continue to care. When we practice by relational ethics grounded in a solution-focused approach, we are not practicing solely by policy, procedure, or routine. This type of practice allows us to focus on something that can continue to be worked with and manipulated therapeutically: the relationship with the patient. The notion of *nurses making a difference* requires us to think about areas of practice that are open to our influence. When concrete elements of a situation, such as a diagnosis or a certain course of treatment cannot be changed, we need to think in new and creative ways about how we can work with the patient and how we can be a useful resource for them.

CONCLUSION

Wherever nursing care is provided, there is the possibility, even the likelihood, of limitations either to the caring itself or to the environment in which the care is provided. We cannot always achieve everything we and our patients may hope for in the caring encounter. Furthermore, we do not always practice in ideal environments, in which, all necessary resources are at our disposal. Nurses need ways to transcend or manage these limitations to stay relevant, both for the patient and in the wider arena of health care provision.

Nursing is regulated by professional bodies that set standards for practice and ethical conduct. As we practise according to these standards, we reflect upon and analyse our actions in an attempt to improve the care that we provide. Solution-focused, relational ethics assists us to practice within professional frameworks, despite limitations, by helping us to appraise "what is" occurring in practice and thinking about transforming that practice into what "could be." By striving for that which could be, nurses are not settling for practice that is "safe" or "good enough." Striving to situate ourselves morally in the world of our patients and recognising and valuing their place in our world make our practice ethical.

LEARNING ACTIVITIES

1. **A reflection on moral practice.** Have you experienced what Jameton (1984) termed as "moral distress"? What was the situation and what did you do? You might like to make some reflective notes on this situation that you can revisit as you reread this chapter.
2. **Pairing ethics and the "doing" of nursing.** What influences the ways that you know are the "right things" to do when caring

for patients? What ethical principles have helped in this regard? What else might assist you to be confident in yourself as an ethical practitioner?

3. **Creating forward movement.** Think about a time when you have experienced moral distress, how might a solution-focused ethics has changed the way you approached the situation? What strategies or resources might be useful for you to practice relationally and simultaneously fulfill your obligations to your professional code of conduct?

4. **Final food for thought.** Consider this quote from the Roman Stoic philosopher Marcus Aurelius (trans. 1997), "You've wandered all over and finally realised that you never found what you were after: how to live." What sort of changes in ethical thinking does it imply? How do you want to "live" as a nurse?

REFERENCES

Aurelius, M. (1997). *Meditations* (R. Hard, Trans.). Hertfordshire, UK: Wordsworth Editions Limited.

Austin, W., Kelecevic, J., Goble, E., & Mekechuk, J. (2009). An overview of moral distress and the pediatric intensive care team. *Nursing Ethics, 16*(1), 57–68. doi: 10.1177/0969733008097990

Benedict, S., & Kuhla, J. (1999). Nurses' participation in the euthanasia programs of Nazi Germany. *Western Journal of Nursing Research, 21*(2), 246–263. doi: 10.1177/01939459922043749

Gilligan, C. (1982). *In a different voice: Psychological theory and women's development.* Cambridge, MA: Harvard University Press.

Greenfield, B., & Banja, J. (2009). The role of ethical theory in ethical education for physical therapist students. *Journal of Physical Therapy Education, 23* (2), 24–28.

Jameton, A. (1984). *Nursing practice: The ethical issues.* Englewood Cliffs, NJ: Prentice Hall.

Kant, I. (1949). *The philosophy of Kant: Immanuel Kant's moral and political writings.* New York, NY: Modern Library.

Kant, I. (2002). *Critique of practical reason* (W. S. Pluhar, Trans.). Indianapolis, IN: Hackett Publishing. (Original work published 1788)

McAllister, M. (2007). *Solution focused nursing: Rethinking practice.* Basingstoke, UK: Palgrave Macmillan.

Nelson, H. L. (2000). Feminist bioethics: Where we've been, where we're going. *Metaphilosophy, 31*(5), 492–508. doi: 10.1111/1467-9973.00165

Nelson, S., & Gordon, S. (Eds.). (2006). *The complexities of care: Nursing reconsidered.* Ithaca, NY: Cornell University Press.

Noddings, N. (2003). *Caring: A feminine approach to ethics and moral education* (2nd ed.). Berkeley, CA: University of California Press.

Oberle, K., & Raffin-Bouchal, S. (2009). *Ethics in Canadian nursing practice: Navigating the journey.* Toronto, Canada: Pearson Education Canada.

Slote, M. (2007). *The ethics of care and empathy.* Abingdon, UK: Routledge.

(4) Learning From Role Models

Maura MacPhee

INTRODUCTION

Human beings learn in various ways, and numerous learning theories have attempted to understand and develop best ways for people to acquire or adapt behaviours, values, and attitudes conducive to a productive life (e.g., see Erikson, 1968; Gardner, 1983; Pavlov, 1927; Vygotsky, 1978). According to one such theory, known as social learning theory (Bandura, 1997), we learn best through others. The focus for this chapter is to introduce to you the idea of using aspects of social learning theory to empower your practice.

THE STORY

Imagine yourself as a new graduate nurse on a busy acute care surgery unit. You have come prepared. You have your stethoscope, nursing scissors, and tape roll. In your locker, you store an extra set of scrubs and some toiletries. Your lunch is stored safely in the staff fridge, and you are ready for report. Your preceptor meets you at the nursing station. She is a registered nurse with 6 years experience on the unit. She immediately puts you at ease. She says, "I'm really looking forward to working with you. I've oriented other new staff, and I really enjoy teaching." She does quick team introductions. Everybody is welcoming towards you, including the nursing manager.

After report and patient rounds with your team, your preceptor reviews the day's schedule with you. She explains that she has already met with the educator to design an orientation plan to familiarise you with procedures specific to the unit and to gradually increase your independence.

You make several observations on this day. You notice a nurse talking with one of the surgeons about a patient's discharge plan. This nurse seems professional, confident, and respectful. He also advocates for the patient and her family. You admire his articulate manner. A certified wound care nurse invites you to watch her do a dressing change. During the dressing change, she doesn't just act; she explains everything she is doing. You consider that her "think-out-loud" style effectively reassures the patient and provides evidence-based rationales for her actions that help you to remember the principles. Again, you admire her proficiency and make a mental note to explain your actions to patients in future.

Towards the end of the shift, your preceptor and you debrief about what you noticed, and what you would like to learn more about. The preceptor finishes the interaction by saying, "Thank you for giving your best today. You really pitched in, you asked some great questions, and you were kind and caring towards the patients."

As you walk out the door, you take a moment to consider how you feel. You realise that apart from feeling tired and thirsty, you are feeling more confident and comfortable with your colleagues, and you are looking forward to returning tomorrow. You think you can do this!

THE POWER OF SOCIAL LEARNING

Social learning theory says that we can learn by observation, imitation, and role modelling (Bandura, 1997). But learning isn't guaranteed, and it isn't automatic. Bandura (1997) explained that sometimes, this learning can occur quite subtly, or implicitly, without your conscious attention, as if through osmosis. However, we learn most from observing others when we (a) pay close attention, (b) attempt to remember and retain what we thought worthwhile, (c) reproduce those observed behaviours later as a kind of trial emulation, and (d) have the motivation to acquire these observed behaviours—if there's no pay off (such as becoming a better nurse), then it's unlikely that we will learn from others, even if their actions are effective.

Two key resiliency skills for nurses: find a good role model and then be a good role model for others.

You can also learn in the absence of real-life social interaction. For example, nursing students may learn a procedure by watching a video demonstration and may pick up basic knowledge and skills about performing a procedure, but something important is lacking from this learning process. The missing element is the web of social interaction that is possible when learning occurs with others. In these interactions, you can observe and ask questions to clarify uncertainties, and the demonstrator can repeat an action or explain something further. The learning that can occur in conversation and in interaction with others is more complex and rich, and gives you greater opportunities to notice, retain, and practice the action under guidance than learning in isolation does. This social learning process, between you and experienced nurses, will do more than build your competence with respect to knowledge and skills. It will also build your confidence, or what psychologists call "personal efficacy." Personal efficacy is the belief in the self.

REALITY SHOCK

The story provided presented an ideal situation—one in which the preceptor had an opportunity to prepare for your arrival and customise a learning experience for you. The story included at least three positive observational learning experiences and, being the astute learner that you are, you not only noticed them, you did the mental work necessary to remember them because you were motivated and thoughtful. Situations won't always be positive and you won't always have the energy and awareness to notice, filter, and retain only the most effective practices.

In addition, with current nursing shortages, experienced preceptors are not always available. With the busyness of most health care settings, new graduates often have to "hit the ground running," even if they aren't familiar with the unit staff, layout, or specific practices.

Also, you may see less than ideal practice—in which interactions aren't effective, people don't communicate well and standards are not maintained. You may see nurses practising out of habit or routine, rather than best evidence. You may see tempers flare when patients do not have their needs met, and staff members become impatient, frustrated, and rude under the pressures of modern workplaces. You may also encounter generational, racial, gender, or power conflicts, and you may be tested and expected to earn credibility. All of this can add up to reality shock.

> Reality shock will have less impact if you are prepared for being the new kid who has more questions than answers, distress in clients and families, and interpersonal tension within the team. How will you respond to these issues in ways that ease tension and avoid blame?

How close to your ideals is the reality of practice depends on unit culture. A unit's culture is shaped by the people in the unit and how they choose to interact with each other. The culture reflects the values of the unit members (Tanner, 2006). If you experience a negative nursing culture in which your professional ideals are different from the values of those around you, reality shock can erode your confidence and your commitment to be a nurse (Young, Stuenkel, & Bawel-Brinkley, 2008).

Health care workplaces use various strategies to diminish reality shock for new graduates. Some of them were mentioned in the story—a formal orientation period, provision of an experienced preceptor, close supervision by a manager or educator, and the opportunity to reflect or debrief. These formal strategies are meant to promote learning and socialise you to the profession (Cowin & Hengstberger-Sims, 2006). Their effectiveness depends on the quality of the relationship between the graduate and others and on the astuteness and motivation of the graduate for learning and self-efficacy.

In one research study in the United States, graduate nurses in their first year of practice were interviewed about those factors that helped them successfully transition from school to practice (Zinsmeister & Schafer, 2009). They identified five factors that helped them most: a supportive work environment, a good preceptor, comprehensive orientation, concrete role expectations, and a solid core of values and belief in oneself. Thus, successfully overcoming reality shock is a collaborative process that depends on your work colleagues, the unit culture—and you.

BECOMING AN EFFECTIVE NURSE

Becoming a confident, effective nurse is a socialisation process that takes time. Socialisation is how we pass on our professional roles and responsibilities from experienced nurses to graduate nurses (Godinez, Schweiger, Gruver, & Ryan, 1999). Typically, it takes 18 months to 2 years for a new nurse to feel comfortable in the role, become clinically competent, and establish a confident nursing identity (Benner, 1984; Schoessler & Waldo, 2006).

Part of this socialisation process involves a period of accommodation in which the mismatch between reality and ideals evens out. However, graduates who are not aware of this settling-in period may become impatient, frustrated, disillusioned, and disheartened by the differences between the ideal and the reality that they experience. Many new nurses simply give up and leave (Casey, Fink, Krugman, & Propst, 2004). Aside from simply being aware that accommodation takes time, a useful strategy to empower your practice during this period is to identify your "must haves" (nonnegotiable ideals) and distinguish them from the "nice to haves" (negotiable ideals). This strategy can be enacted and reenacted throughout your career as your values, needs, and aspirations change.

Although the socialisation process starts in school, your first work environments will probably have the biggest influence on you. If you are open to the experiences and mindful of the four elements explained at the beginning of this chapter as maximising the power of social learning, your confidence will grow. You will be on a steep learning curve—acquiring skilful practices, knowledge of services and key people, know-how with patients, repartee with colleagues, and sound clinical judgment. As Schoessler and Waldo (2006) stated, "each day in practice is another day of learning and another day closer to competent practice" (p. 49). But remember that this isn't an automatic process. Simple exposure to skilful practices or positive role models is no guarantee that graduates will acquire the same proficiency: It takes conscious intent on the part of the learner.

Critical thinking is also important because there will be many times when you will need to discern which practices you wish to model and those that you believe would not fit well with your values and aspirations in the long term (du Toit, 1995; Young et al., 2008). Thus, to extend Bandura's theory, we suggest that for you to take charge of your professional development, you need to have motivation and to practise attention, retention, imitative practice, and discernment.

A key strategy to empower your practice: become discerning about the people and practices you observe and emulate.

SELF-EFFICACY

Bandura's social learning theory has now been extended, tested, and applied by many researchers and, whilst studies vary, strong evidence now demonstrates that personal self-efficacy is key to achieving positive change (e.g., see Lorig, 2003; Strachan & Brawley, 2009; Wangberg, 2008). Knowledge and skills are important, but self-efficacy is the strongest predictor of actual success (Bandura, 2004); many people with average skills have surpassed individuals with great talent because of their strong belief in themselves.

Personal efficacy develops when the learner is socially engaged. Conversely, a lack of self-belief, disengagement from social learning experiences, and lack of attention lead to failure to learn.

A lack of self-belief, disengagement from the learning experience, and lack of attention lead to failure to learn.

This key insight is relevant not only to yourself as a lifelong learner but also for your work with patients. If patients and their significant others are not ready, willing, or able to observe the things you are trying to model, they won't retain the information. Also, if they don't believe they are capable, learning and change are unlikely to occur. Spending time preparing patients to build up their self-efficacy and concentration, in addition to maximising the learning experience, will be empowering strategies for you and for them (Lorig, 2000).

EFFECTIVE ROLE MODELLING

Allanach (1988) provides a useful feedback cycle to apply with role models and modellers, the "competence–confidence feedback cycle." This feedback loop exists between an experienced nurse role model and a new nurse when feedback is provided during every demonstration of competence, thus growing confidence within the new nurse. This feedback loop is also more likely to result in successful transition to practice. Reflect on our original story and find examples in which this cycle was used and, perhaps, other instances with potential to use it. Remembering to use this feedback cycle is another important strategy to empower your practice as you become a role model for others.

In addition to the competence–confidence building that occurs with regular constructive feedback, something else also happens in the relationship with a role model. Because this is a social process, you will start to learn more about your role model, and your role model will learn about you. You may develop an emotional relationship that will add to your confidence and reinforce positive values (Godinez et al., 1999). We tend to build these affective bonds with role models who share our values (Jordan & Farley, 2009). You can probably recall situations at school or university where you "clicked" with some teachers and not with others. This happens with role models as well. You will no doubt encounter many experienced nurses who will advance your knowledge and skills, but you will probably only develop emotional ties with those role models who match your values.

These value connections are important in developing personal efficacy. In a recent study with new midwifery graduates, the graduates were asked to complete surveys about their values, their perceptions of their preceptors' values, and their level of personal efficacy (Jordan & Farley, 2009). A perception of similar values was significantly associated with new graduates' self-confidence or efficacy.

Here are some qualities that Australian nursing students identified as great values in role models: caring, respectfulness, having a positive attitude about service or care delivery, and moral integrity (du Toit, 1995). It's important to have role models who can build your personal efficacy through regular guidance and feedback and who share a conviction about the value and importance of nursing.

> Key strategy to empower your practice: clarify your values about nursing, then find role models who share your values.

You will have many role models throughout your life, but as you transition from new graduate nurse to competent nurse, it's important that you have consistent, experienced nurse role models. Consistency is necessary for you to get to know each other. Many health care organisations make concerted efforts to establish orientation programs in which new graduates have a few consistent preceptors (Paton, Thompson-Isherwood, & Thirsk, 2009). Consistent preceptors will have a better idea of how to structure learning opportunities for you, clarify your role responsibilities, and support your gradual independence (Casey et al., 2004; Zinsmeister & Schafer, 2009). In one U.S. study, new graduate nurses felt that their orientation went more smoothly when they had no more than three preceptors (Casey et al., 2004). In today's complex health care settings, preceptor coordination during orientation may prove difficult. In instances in which you may have to work with multiple preceptors, a nurse manager or educator can oversee your orientation and ensure learning continuity across different preceptors (Casey et al., 2004).

Many health care settings have preceptor programs because effective preceptors increase retention of new nurses (Hickey, 2009; Paton et al., 2009). Preceptors often volunteer to work with new nurses because they enjoy teaching, and research has shown that preceptors derive satisfaction from supporting the professional growth and development of new nurses (Neumann et al., 2004; Wright, 2002). In addition, preceptors often experience increased personal efficacy by acting as role models for new nurses (Canadian Nurses Association, 2004).

The Canadian Nurses Association (2004) developed a list of preceptor competencies based on research evidence in nursing (Table 4.1). The competencies encompass knowledge, skills, and attitudes. These competencies are successful ingredients for preceptors and for nurse role models in general. Consider the table and reflect on the values and behaviours that you would add, based on your student experiences.

You will notice that one of the competencies under *"Professional Practice"* is described as "clinically proficient." We know from research that some of the best preceptors and role models for new nurses are clinically proficient nurses (Uhrenfeldt & Hall, 2007; Valdez, 2008). Clinically proficient nurses are clinically wise nurses. Their actions are firmly connected to critical thinking and ethical judgment (Benner, Tanner, & Chesla, 2009; Uhrenfeldt & Hall, 2007). In a Danish study that explored the characteristics of proficient nurses, these nurses remained calm as they carefully evaluated their care options and, most importantly, they focused on their patient's concerns (Uhrenfeldt & Hall, 2007). To become this type of nurse takes time and practice, but the good news for you is that there are many proficient nurses out there!

TABLE 4.1   Canadian Nurses Association Preceptor Competencies (2004)

Preceptor Competency	Description
Collaboration	Collaborates with learners, colleagues, manager/educators, patients
Personal attributes	Enthusiastic, flexible, respectful, self-confident, good listener and communicator
Facilitation of learning	Identifies and plans individualised learning opportunities; provides ongoing constructive feedback; intervenes immediately in unsafe and unethical situations; asks open-ended questions to gain a better understanding of the learner; provides reinforcement by focusing on learner strengths
Professional practice	Consistently upholds nursing standards of practice and code of ethics; current in evidence-based practice; clinically proficient
Knowledge of the setting	Knows the organisation's vision and mission, systems of care, policies and procedures, learning resources, who's who, the physical layout

ROLE MODELS: WHERE YOU MAY FIND THEM

Health care organisations often appoint nurses as preceptors when they are considered proficient or able to effectively perceive the entirety of the clinical situation (Valdez, 2008). In addition to preceptor programs, various other programs such as internships and mentoring programs have been credited with successfully transitioning new graduates (Blanzola, Lindeman, & King, 2004; Canadian Nurses Association, 2004; Newhouse, Hoffman, Suflita, & Hairtson, 2007). The critical component in all these programs is effective nurse role models. You may be fortunate to obtain your first job at an organisation that promotes some or all of these wonderful programs for new graduates, but if not, you can always identify your own role models.

Check out your institution's nurse managers and educators. They are generally in formal positions of authority because of their ability to lead others, their clinical competence, and their knowledge of the practice environment (Valdez, 2008). They will also know how to get you started and how to keep you on track because they are invested in your success: They have recruited you and they want to retain you as part of their staff. They will know the frustrations and stressors out there, and they will do their best to buffer your entry into practice. This is a two-way process though, and you will need to set up regular meetings with them in which you can review your progress and be honest about your concerns and needs.

Other good prospects for role models are nurses certified with specialties, clinical nurse specialists, or advanced practice nurses who care for specific patient populations because of their clinical proficiency or expertise. An example is the wound care nurse in our story. During your orientation, get to know these resource people. Look through the institution's directory and locate nurses with specific specialties. Make an effort to connect with these nurses because they often spend a good portion of their time with patients, planning care collaboratively and teaching patients how to improve their health and well- being. If you observe them in action, you will learn some great patient-centred strategies such as the think-out-loud strategy mentioned in the story. Thinking out loud reveals the problem-solving process, including the use of research evidence (Reilly, 2007). You should cultivate this technique for yourself, and it's a definite bonus to find experienced nurse role models who will think out loud for you.

Where else will you find good role models? Go back to our story for some other clues. During shift reports and patient care rounds, you may identify similar nurses who model evidence-based practice, assertive communication, client advocacy, and holistic nursing practice (Ferguson & Day, 2007). Listen and observe: Some nurses will emerge as critical thinkers and patient advocates. Interdisciplinary team meetings, such as discharge planning meetings or patient care conferences are other places to look for effective role models. You may even find some non–nurse role models who personify the values and beliefs you have about professional health care delivery. Some of my first role models were a pharmacist, a respiratory therapist, and a physician. What were my "must-have" values? On the top of my list were compassionate care and evidence-based practice.

Nurses will certainly have a major influence over your professional socialisation, and you will have many opportunities to listen to and observe them during shift report and rounds, even in the staff lounge. Be courageous. Engage in conversations with them and listen to their stories. We know that having and telling stories about practice experiences is an important way in which nurses turn their experiences into practical knowledge and understanding (Tanner, 2006). Nurses often reveal their values through the stories they tell (Forneris & Peden-McAlpine, 2006). By listening and asking questions, many rich stories will unfold around you. Do you feel value connections with particular nurses? Turn to these nurses during times of ethical or moral turmoil when you need to talk through a dilemma and sort out your values (Yancy, 2005).

WHAT MORE CAN YOU DO?

As you enter the practice environment as a new nurse, you may be filled with a mix of elation and anxiety. These are normal feelings and many other new nurses will be facing similar hopes and fears (Schoessler & Waldo, 2006). Be sure to focus on your positives: You've made it. Take stock of what you've already accomplished before you start your first job, and share your joy in these accomplishments with your manager, the educator, and your preceptor. There's nothing wrong with sharing your pride in hard-won achievements and it also demonstrates that you are hardworking and self-motivated. These qualities are admirable in any worker.

Reflect on your strengths. You probably know how to provide basic care for many of the patients on the unit and you, no doubt, have a grasp of the common medications and procedures. What else can you do and what else do you know? Are you organised, outgoing, and optimistic? Let others know what strengths you bring to your new practice environment—it's certainly more productive than focusing on what you cannot do!

Connect with other new nurses because they can be a great source of support for you. In one U.S. orientation program, new nurses participated in regular scheduled discussions. Each discussion ranged from 2 to 3 hours in which orientees networked among themselves and talked about issues of patient care with advanced practice nurses. These discussions provided exposure to experienced role models and to other graduates' insights about the successes and challenges related to the socialisation process. Nurse researchers compared the graduates of this program to new nurses who did not have this orientation experience (Blanzola et al., 2004). Program participants had improved levels of confidence in their ability to succeed, even in complex care situations. If formal peer group sessions do not exist in your first job setting, you can always create your own informal support network. Peer networks offer camaraderie, a sounding board for common issues, and, potentially, a source of peer role models—new nurses, like you, who have found successful strategies for transitioning into practice. You may even serve as a role model for your peers!

CONCLUSION

Socialisation is a lifelong process. According to social learning theory, our role models influence whom we become. We can increase the power of social learning by being observant, making a conscious effort to remember the things we've just learned through the role model, practising the observed behaviour in the way that we saw it, and believing in ourselves and our roles as nurses.

This chapter has provided you with several strategies drawn from social learning theory that can empower your practice. I've offered you examples of the characteristics of successful role models from research around the world and discussed where you can find good role models. Now it's up to you to find the motivation, self-belief, and effective role models to help you achieve your nursing goals.

LEARNING ACTIVITIES

1. Generate class discussion on the value of knowing the self. Ask learners to make a list of their "must-have" and "nice-to-have" employment conditions. Ask learners to discuss how they intend to bridge the divide between the ideals and the reality of practice.
2. Students can complete this webquest in their own time or take 20 minutes of computer-based learning during class.
3. Think of a health care organisation for which you might want to work after graduation. Check out its website. Highlight key words that stand out for you in the organisation's vision, mission, or value statement. Do you identify with these highlighted words? It is important to choose a place to work with values that match your values.

4. Look at the website for a professional nursing organisation such as the Canadian Nurses Association, or the Royal College of Nursing, Australia. What key nursing values stand out for you as you look at the site? Do you agree with the way that professional nursing is portrayed on the site? Why or why not?
5. Drawing on individual or group "must haves," construct a role model checklist to help learners become discerning about the colleagues they choose as positive role models.

REFERENCES

Allanach, B. (1988). Interviewing to evaluate preceptorship relationships. *Journal for Nurses in Staff Development, 4*(4), 152–157.

Bandura, A. (1997). *Self-efficacy: The exercise of control.* New York, NY: W. H. Freeman and Company.

Bandura, A. (2004). Health promotion by social cognitive means. *Health Education and Behavior, 31*(2), 143–164.

Benner, P. (1984). *From novice to expert: Excellence and power in clinical nursing practice.* Menlo Park, CA: Addison-Wesley Publishing.

Benner, P., Tanner, C., & Chesla, C. (2009). *Expertise in nursing practice: Caring, clinical judgment, and ethics* (2nd ed.). New York, NY: Springer.

Blanzola, C., Lindeman, R., & King, L. (2004). Nurse internship pathway to clinical comfort, confidence, and competency. *Journal for Nurses in Staff Development, 20*(1), 27–37.

Canadian Nurses Association. (2004). *Achieving excellence in professional practice—a guide to preceptorship and mentoring.* Retrieved from http://www.cna-nurses.ca/CNA/documents/pdf/publications/Achieving_Excellence_2004_e.pdf

Casey, K., Fink, R., Krugman, M., & Propst, J. (2004). The graduate nurse experience. *Journal of Nursing Administration, 34*(6), 303–311.

Cowin, L., & Hengstberger-Sims, C. (2006). New graduate nurse self-concept and retention: A longitudinal survey. *International Journal of Nursing Studies, 43*, 59–70.

du Toit, D. (1995). A sociological analysis of the extent and influence of professional socialization on the development of a nursing identity among nursing students at two universities in Brisbane, Australia. *Journal of Advanced Nursing, 21*(1), 164–171.

Erikson, E. (1968). *Identity: Youth and crisis.* New York, NY: Norton.

Ferguson, L., & Day, R. (2007). Challenges for new nurses in evidence-based practice. *Journal of Nursing Management, 15*, 107-113.

Forneris, S., & Peden-McAlpine, C. (2006). Contextual learning: A reflective learning intervention for nursing education. *International Journal of Nursing Education Scholarship, 3*(1), 1-18. Retrieved from CINAHL database.

Gardner, H. (1983). *Frames of mind: The theory of multiple intelligences.* New York, NY: Basic Books.

Godinez, G., Schweiger, J., Gruver, J., & Ryan, P. (1999). Role transition from graduate to staff nurse: A qualitative analysis. *Journal for Nurses in Staff Development, 15*(3), 97-110.

Hickey, M. (2009). Preceptor perceptions of new graduate nurse readiness to practice. *Journal for Nurses in Staff Development, 25*(1), 35-41.

Jordan, R., & Farley, C. (2009). The confidence to practice midwifery: Preceptor influence on student self-efficacy. *Journal of Midwifery and Women's Health, 53*(5), 413-420.

Lorig, K. (2000). *Patient education: A practical approach* (3rd ed.). New York, NY: Sage Publications.

Lorig, K. (2003). Self-management education. More than a nice extra. *Medical Care, 41*(6), 699-701.

Neumann, J., Brady-Schluttner, K., McKay, A., Roslien, J., Twedell, D., & James, K. (2004). Centralizing a registered nurse preceptor program at an institutional level. *Journal for Nurses in Staff Development, 20*(1), 17-24.

Newhouse, R., Hoffman, J., Suflita, J., & Hairtson, D. (2007). Evaluating an innovative program to improve new nurse graduate socialization into the acute care setting. *Nursing Administration Quarterly, 31*(1), 50-60.

Paton, B., Thompson-Isherwood, R., & Thirsk, L. (2009). Preceptors matter: An evolving framework. *Journal of Nursing Education, 48*(4), 213-216.

Pavlov, I. (1927). *Conditioned reflexes: An investigation of the physiological activity of the cerebral cortex.* Translated and edited by G. V. Anrep. London: Oxford University Press.

Reilly, B. (2007). Inconvenient truths about effective clinical teaching. *The Lancet, 370*(9588), 705-711.

Schoessler, M., & Waldo, M. (2006). The first 18 months in practice: A developmental transition model for the newly graduated nurse. *Journal for Nurses in Staff Development, 22*(2), 47-52.

Strachan, S., & Brawley, L. (2009). Healthy-eater identity and self-efficacy predict healthy eating behavior: A prospective view. *Journal of Health Psychology, 14*(5), 684-695.

Tanner, C. (2006). Thinking like a nurse: A research-based model of clinical judgment in nursing. *Journal of Nursing Education, 45*(6), 204-211.

Uhrenfeldt, L., & Hall, E. (2007). Clinical wisdom among proficient nurses. *Nursing Ethics, 14*(3), 387-398.

Valdez, A. M. (2008). Transitioning from novice to competent: What can we learn from the literature about graduate nurses in the emergency setting? *Journal of Emergency Nursing, 34*(5), 435–440.

Vygotsky, L. (1978). *Mind and society: The development of higher mental processes.* Cambridge, MA: Harvard University Press.

Wangberg, S. (2008). An Internet-based diabetes self-care intervention tailored to self-efficacy. *Health Education Research, 23*(1), 170–179.

Wright, A. (2002). Preceptoring in 2002. *The Journal for Continuing Education in Nursing, 33*(3), 138–141.

Yancy, N. (2005). The experience of the novice nurse: A human becoming perspective. *Nursing Science Quarterly, 18*(3), 215–220.

Young, M., Stuenkel, D., & Bawel-Brinkley, K. (2008). Strategies for easing the role transformation of graduate nurses. *Journal for Nurses in Staff Development, 24*(3), 105–110.

Zinsmeister, L., & Schafer, D. (2009). The exploration of the lived experience of the graduate nurse making the transition to registered nurse during the first year of practice. *Journal for Nurses in Staff Development, 25*(1), 28–34.

Thinking Clearly: Realistic Appraisals and Moderating Reactions in Stressful Situations

Mary Katsikitis and Rachael R. Sharman

INTRODUCTION

We all encounter stressful situations in our daily work life. But how does the way we perceive, or think about, these situations affect our reactions? Success in any profession requires an ability to make clear judgements and to moderate our "natural" response to a stressful encounter. In this chapter, we will discuss the influence of appraisals—the judgements we make—during a stressful scenario and how these appraisals might affect our reactions under stress. We will compare and contrast the functional impact of different appraisal and reactive styles, particularly in terms of how your perceptions and judgements affect both you and those around you. The focus will be on learning to identify and, perhaps, modify our own patterns of thinking and psychological approaches. We will also provide some tips on how to moderate your reactions under stress to make clearer judgements and conduct yourself in a professional manner that benefits everyone.

THE STORY

It is your first day on a new rotation. You are nervous because you've heard rumours that this is a "difficult" ward to work in. You are eager to make a good first impression, but the day does not start well. You have difficulty finding a car park and did not realise that the parking, even for staff, would be so crowded and expensive! As you rush to the ward to which you've been assigned, you quickly become lost in the labyrinth of corridors and suddenly, you realise that you will be lucky to arrive on time. You are feeling pressured and frustrated, and your heart is racing. You arrive and introduce yourself to the nurse unit manager with apologies for your lateness and are immediately relieved when the manager sympathises with your parking drama and your difficulty in finding the ward. The manager offers to show you around and introduces you to the staff present on the ward. Most of the staff members seem friendly and pleasant. Although a little preoccupied with their tasks at hand, they briefly stop to smile, shake your hand, and welcome you to the ward. You start to relax a little and begin to look forward to the day ahead. Suddenly, a physician strides quickly into the area. The physician looks angry. A few orders are barked at another nurse across the other side of the room, about a patient in Room 3. The physician leans over the main counter, snatches a medical file, and proceeds to read it intently. You stand there saying nothing, not knowing what to do, and you notice your heart is beating fast again. Suddenly, the physician looks up, notices you, turns to the unit manager, and asks, "Who's this?" The manager politely introduces the physician as the "doctor in charge" and introduces you as the new trainee nurse. Unlike everyone else, the physician makes no move to acknowledge you at all, just looks back at the medical file and *sighs*, "Oh, fantastic!"

How do you feel about this exchange? How do you interpret the physician's behaviour, sigh, and comment? Is the physician pleased to have you on the ward today, or are you just another nuisance in the already hectic schedule? What is your immediate response to this situation? Are you thrilled that the physician has given a sigh of relief and that your presence here today is "fantastic"? Do you sympathise with the physician for having a bad day? Do you interpret the sigh and comment as a sarcastic gesture, but shrug off the remark? Or, can you already feel tears welling in your eyes and a rising feeling of dread about your new job?

You may be surprised to learn that your interpretation and reaction to this situation may have more to do with your current physiological state and some inbuilt personal thinking styles, rather than an objective analysis of what has just occurred. Any of these reactions may be considered—by different people—to be totally justified under the circumstances. How *you* think and feel about any situation is a highly individual process. However, let's take each of the preceding different reactive styles to their logical conclusions to assess the impact each will have on you and the people around you.

How you interpret situations may have more to do with your personal thinking styles than the event itself.

THE FUNCTIONAL IMPACT OF REACTIVE STYLES

An important thing to consider is how would each of these very different reactions mentioned earlier affect both your functioning and the functioning of the people around you? The following exercise analyses the *functional impact* of each reactive style.

1. You are thrilled that the doctor has indicated your presence here today is "fantastic!" Now, some of you will have baulked as soon as you read this—totally disbelieving that anyone would have interpreted the situation in this way. Well, all we can say is—you are wrong! There are a group of individuals in our population who have what psychologists call an *optimistic explanatory style* (Peterson, 2000). Like any reactive style, this one has its strengths and weaknesses (Tennen & Affleck, 1987). These are the people who happily take credit for their successes but minimise their personal involvement in any failures. They tend to filter information in a very self-protective manner, ignoring negative feedback and maximising positive feedback (Lazarus, 1983; Martin-Krumm, Sarrazin, Peterson, & Famose, 2003). Before you assume that these people are all delusional or narcissistic (and it's no surprise, this style is highly correlated with both!), in most (mild-to-moderate) cases, this style makes for a fairly functional person (Martin-Krumm et al., 2003; Taylor & Brown, 1988). These people interpret everything in the most positive light possible and are almost impossible to offend. They may be viewed by colleagues as mildly deranged for their overly optimistic response to absolutely everything, or perhaps even a bit "full of themselves." However, their confidence, sunny dispositions, and thick hides make them enjoyable and often fun to have around. The major downside to people with this reactive style is that they can be insensitive to the needs or the state of those around them. This person may be the one who responds to the physician's comment by slapping him on the back and saying, "Great to be here too, Doc!" The person may then try to engage the physician in further conversation despite it being obvious that he has other pressing things on his mind. They're not trying to be sarcastic or funny; they just assume that everyone thinks well of them. They can therefore be insensitive to the negative signals coming from others and react inappropriately at times.

2. You sympathise with the physician and assume he is having a bad day. This kind of reaction is known as an *external attribution* towards the physician. The focus is taken off you and placed squarely back on the doctor. People who react in this way interpret the situation as being largely about the physician's situational factors. Hence, they are likely to feel empathy and compassion for the physician's needs, rather than take offence that their own needs have been violated in any way. They also deflect any negative self-view in this way and, in doing so, often project kindness towards others that is usually noticed and well received. People who react in this manner may be said to "take the high road" and, again, are usually valued as thoughtful and kind employees in the workplace. Happily, they also suffer little negative emotion towards themselves—after all, the physician is having the bad day, not them!

3. You interpret the physician's remark as sarcastic, but shrug it off. In this case, you have made an *internal attribution* towards the physician's motives—perhaps, he is a bad-tempered person or has no manners. Now, on the face of it, this seems like a fairly functional response. But think again: Even if you casually shrug off the comment, you have interpreted some small level of malice in the physician's response to you. People who react in this way may, in the future, dislike or even avoid this physician. They may engage in the silent treatment or use a terse manner towards the physician until they receive an apology. Their thinking at this moment may take the following form: "The physician is being sarcastic; the physician is rude; the physician is being horrible to me and I've done nothing to deserve this, but I'm just going to ignore it because the physician is just an arrogant." So, whilst the immediate effect on those around you is neutral (you don't obviously respond one way or the other), the functional impact of this response on *you* is likely to be negative. This negative impact may then continue to influence how you deal

with this person in the future, and you are likely to harbour some malice towards them.

4. You feel tears welling and a feeling of dread about your new job. This reactive style is probably the most dysfunctional, both for you and for the people around you. However, this style is very common especially among younger people who tend to be a lot more self-conscious (you learn to care a lot less about what other people think of you as you get older!). People with this reactive style are interpreting the event as being all about them, rather than being about the physician's manner or his current circumstances. Psychologists call this a *pessimistic explanatory style* (Dykema, Bergbower, & Peterson, 1995) and, over time, people with this reactive style tend to have impaired job performance, more physical illness, and more social distress (Jackson, Sellers, & Peterson, 2002; Peterson, Seligman, & Vaillant, 1988). Think about this reaction for a moment. You feel distressed and offended, and if others perceive the tears welling in your eyes, they feel upset for you. The unit manager may react initially with surprise, but then try to reassure you. The physician may apologise, but conversely, he may become quite irritated with your reaction. If the physician's comment was meant kindly, he may even take offence at your reaction! Any way you look at it, the functional impact of your behaviour, if you react in this manner, is to take everyone's focus off his or her job and place it squarely onto you. This reactive style, for obvious reasons, is the one least valued in workplaces. Work colleagues learn they have to worry about your reactions, perhaps "walk around on egg shells" and take valuable time out of their hectic schedules to deal with you. Furthermore, and worst of all, *you* feel awful—very much a lose–lose situation!

Evaluating and Moderating Your Reactive Style

When you find yourself feeling, thinking, and reacting in a particular way, ask yourself these questions: What purpose does this reaction serve? How does this reaction make me feel? How does it affect my functioning? What is the likely effect of this reaction on those around me (both positive and negative)? Try to think of the functional effects of your reaction; in essence, what will be achieved by reacting this way?

Now, if we could moderate our emotions easily and shift our reactions to this- or-that style, there would be none of the wonderful variety in human interaction. So, by no means are we suggesting that you can (or should) always fully control your natural reactive style but at least be prepared to do a double take, to reassess and to reevaluate how you are interpreting and responding to your environment. You may be surprised to find there are ways of changing your perceptions and reactive style, which will also change the way you feel and cope. We will discuss these in the next section.

> The way we perceive and respond to other people is a highly individual trait, usually operating on a continuum from optimistic to pessimistic. Before you react, think about the functional implications of your reaction and ask yourself: How will my response affect me and the people around me? Will my reaction hinder or help?
>
> Which of the four reactions seemed most like you? Can you think of a situation where your reaction changed a situation for the worse? How could you have reacted differently? What do you think the outcome might have been then?

LEARNING TO CHANGE YOUR REACTIVE STYLE

The Impact of Physiological Arousal

Now be honest. Have you ever misinterpreted a situation when you were angry? Perhaps, have you interpreted a harmless comment as a threat or insult? Conversely, have you ever felt wildly attracted to someone during a highly emotional situation? For example, while on holidays, during a stressful work or university project, or while on the rebound from a previous partner? Did you know that your current state of physiological arousal can actually affect your perceptions of your environment and your subsequent emotions?

In 1974, Dutton and Aron conducted an important experiment, often referred to as the "rickety bridge" test. Young men crossed a rickety (it looked dangerous!) bridge to meet an attractive female research assistant, who in turn asked each one a series of questions. The psychologists were interested in whether the high-physiological arousal created in the men (i.e., the fear of crossing the rickety bridge) could then be (mis) attributed by the men as a feeling of desire or lust for the attractive woman. One group of men crossed a stable bridge to meet the assistant whereas the other crossed the rickety bridge. The second group of men, therefore, had their heart and respiratory rates and adrenaline levels raised when they met the attractive young research assistant. The effect of high-physiological arousal on the men's reactions to the research assistant was electrifying. An astoundingly significant four times as many men who crossed the rickety bridge, compared with those who crossed the safe bridge, subsequently made contact with the research assistant to ask her on a date!

Experiments like this one are often used as evidence that we can end up misattributing our current level of physiological arousal to factors in our environment (Pham, 2007; White, Fishbein, & Rutsein, 1981). These men only differed in whether their heart and respiratory rates and adrenaline were elevated when they met the research assistant. The high-arousal group assumed that she was the cause of this feeling and therefore interpreted their physiological arousal, actually caused by the bridge, as being caused by the attractiveness of the female assistant. Such misattribution can, of course, lead us into several errors.

Remember our apprehensive nurse at the beginning of the chapter. She was stressed by her late arrival and expensive car park and was frustrated at getting lost. Her heart rate was up, she was feeling flustered and her physiology was on high alert. Now, how do you think this would have affected her interpretation of the physician's comment? We know from previous research that people in this high-arousal state are much more likely to become defensive or upset, manifested as anger and distress (Rule & Nesdale, 1976; Wild, Clark, Ehlers, & McManus, 2006). As human beings, we are rather obsessed with cause and effect. In other words, if I feel stressed, I want to know what caused it. If a hapless physician marches into my immediate environment and makes an ambiguous comment— bingo! The physician must be the cause of how I'm feeling! Just like the men who misattributed their high level of arousal to the female research assistant, it's alarmingly easy for all of us to make the same error.

Next time you are on "high alert," with your adrenaline racing, be aware that your interpretations of subsequent situations may be coloured by this high-arousal state.

Have you ever been warned not to make a decision while your "blood is boiling," or to "keep a cool head"? This advice is supported by research that indicates decision making is impaired when physiological arousal is high enough to be stressful (Wild et al., 2006). Keinan (1987) found that this impairment mostly resulted from people not assessing all available information; essentially, they jumped to conclusions. In contrast, a moderate level of physiological arousal actually promotes decision making, functioning, and "rising to the challenge" (Seo & Barrett, 2007). But once your physiological arousal gets too high, your brain can interpret the situation as stressful, and anything in your immediate environment can mistakenly be attributed as causing or contributing to that stress.

Health professionals working in hospital settings need to be especially mindful of this effect because they are working in an environment in which many heart-racing moments abound. Anaesthetists, for example, are known to describe their jobs as "99% pure boredom and 1% pure terror," in reference to the usually routine nature of their work, coupled with the rare but potentially fatal complications of anaesthetics. Consider the role of the emergency nurse, midwife, or surgery nurse. All of these professionals are guaranteed some heart-starting and heart-stopping moments in their careers. In these moments, how will your interpretation of events be affected? How might you perceive the interactions with your patients and their caregivers when you are in a stressful situation? Also, how might others in that high state of physiological arousal interpret your actions? Be prepared for unrealistic accusations, threats, and insults to be directed at you when others make erroneous decisions while their "blood is boiling." This may particularly be the case with patients who are undergoing a frightening or even life-threatening procedure.

So what should you do? Firstly, be aware of your current level of arousal and be mindful that it can, and does, affect your interpretation of what's going on around you. When in high arousal, you are predisposed to misinterpret events or comments as threatening or insulting and to react defensively. Sometimes, the best advice in this situation is the oldest: breathe deeply and count to 10 slowly, before you respond. Why has this suggestion stood the test of time? Simple: It is a relaxation technique that will lower your arousal and, by lowering your arousal, you will be able to reappraise your situation with a "cool head." Remember that reactions made in anger and defence can be hard to erase from the memories of those around you or, even worse, they can escalate a bad situation that snowballs into a total catastrophe. In trying to appraise what is going on, ensure that you are in a relaxed state as possible; this strategy will substantially minimise the potentially disastrous errors of judgement that commonly occur in these circumstances.

> Reactions made in anger can be hard to erase from the memories of those around you.

If you are on the receiving end of someone else's misattribution, try not to respond defensively. Instead, calmly restate your position, perhaps giving the other person an opportunity to retreat with dignity. You could make a comment like, "Oh, I'm sorry, I'm not being clear. What I mean is . . . " Once the other person has calmed down, you are likely to receive an apology for the misinterpretation!

Any technique that you can use to relax and return your physiology to normal could be used here. The lesson is, when your blood is boiling, keep your mouth closed. If necessary, debrief after any event in which you thought someone was being unreasonable towards you. Eliciting the opinions of others around you and taking a well-considered approach is much more *functional* than reacting, possibly mistakenly, in a highly emotional moment.

> High-physiological arousal can lead to perceptions of high stress. In trying to uncover the source of our stress, we can mistakenly attribute them to factors in our environment. Nursing practice can provoke very high states of arousal. Remember: When you are at a stressful level of physiological arousal, you are prone to errors in decision making and defensive reactions. Realise that you and your patients are prone to misinterpreting each other's reactions as threatening or insulting during periods of high-physiological arousal. Before responding here, try to calm yourself down or calm your patient down.

Appraisals and Judgements: Changing Your Reactions

Imagine the following scenario: You are tucked up warm in bed on a rainy night. Suddenly, from your comfy bed, you hear a loud bang. You jerk into alertness, your heart races and your breathing quickens. But how do you interpret the bump in the night? And how does that affect the way you react? If you assume that it's the cat jumping off the couch, you will most likely roll over and go straight back to sleep. But what if you interpret the bump as the recently escaped axe murderer trying to get in? Now, how do you feel? Are you inclined to roll over and go back to sleep? No! Your heart rate escalates. Your adrenaline starts pumping and you are preparing to flee or fight. Why? You appraised the bump in the night as danger. In reality, both reactions are equally as silly. In the absence of getting out of bed and checking, you have no real evidence to suggest what caused that bump, although some might argue that the cat is statistically the more likely explanation—assuming you own a cat of course!

The effect of how you *appraise*, or think about, a particular event can markedly alter your interpretation of the event and your reaction to it. Let's go back to our nurse in the story at the beginning. There were four very different appraisals proposed, and each elicited a very different reaction as follows:

1. The nurse takes the physician at her word, appraises the behaviour as welcoming, and takes the comment as a compliment.
2. The nurse appraises the physician as having a bad day and in no way takes the comment personally.
3. The nurse appraises a level of sarcasm in the physician's sigh and comment, does take it personally, but moves on.
4. The nurse appraises the physician's comment as insulting and offensive, takes it personally, and reacts with distress.

The key to moderating our reactions in stressful situations is to attempt to *reappraise* what has happened. We have already discussed the particular importance of this approach if your own physiological level of arousal is high or at stressful levels. Now, we will outline the simple steps you can take to reappraise a situation if you feel you are about to react in a dysfunctional manner (i.e., with anger or distress).

1. Take stock of your own physiology. Are you in a high arousal or stressed state? If so, do nothing in the moment. Instead, leave any response until

later, when you have had a chance to reappraise the situation in a calm and relaxed state. Your likelihood of making an accurate judgement and responding in a functional manner will then be greatly increased.

2. Return again to our nurse–physician interaction. What was your first impression as you read that story? Which response do you think you would most likely have made? So, your next step is to generate as many other "possible appraisals" as you can. The physician has made an ambiguous statement, so what are some other ways you could think about the intent or meaning of that statement? You can actually practise this technique in a range of settings. See the "Learning Activities" for other examples.

3. Seek feedback from others. If, after a calm reappraisal of the evidence, you are still certain that a work colleague or patient is being rude or unreasonable, check with others about their appraisal of the situation. Have you ever said to someone, "Hey, what's wrong with him? Doesn't he like me or something?" Then you are told that the person in question is in terrible circumstances at present, or is battling a health condition, or that he is like that towards everyone, so don't take it personally. This advice can help you to reappraise the scenario and to respond more functionally.

4. If, and only if, it is agreed in a calm and considered manner that someone has, in fact, been unreasonable towards you, what is next? Again, consider the effects of the fourth appraisal and reaction described earlier. In other words, no matter how justified you may be in becoming upset, it's actually not going to help, is it? At this point, a visit to your supervisor may be necessary. You can put forth, in as calm and objective a manner as possible, what happened, what your reaction was (and be honest—own your response, it's your responsibility), and what you think needs to change so you can function better in the environment or situation in future.

Let's now return to our example and talk through the steps that would make for a functional response in this situation. The situation presents itself such that the doctor makes an ambiguous comment while you're in a flustered state. Follow these steps for a resolution that all involved can live with.

1. Acknowledge you are in a high-arousal state and say nothing in the moment. Wait until your physiology has returned to normal to think through the issues.

2. Once you have a "cool head," generate as many reappraisals as you can to explain the physician's response to you. Now that you've calmed down, which one seems most reasonable or most likely?

3. If you're still concerned that what has occurred is unreasonable, seek opinions from others about how *they* perceived the situation, in the most discreet manner possible. You don't want to be accused of being a gossip or a rumour-monger! If you are new, the most appropriate person from whom to seek advice would be the nurse unit manager.

4. Own your personal reactions. In seeking advice, calmly put forth what happened and be very specific about what you found offensive and why. For example, the following explanation could be a specific summary of your thoughts and feelings: *"I got really upset when the physician said that as it was my first day. I was nervous, everyone else was being really nice and I thought what the physician said was rude."*

5. If people agree that what happened is unreasonable, take it to a supervisor for further discussion. It's up to you to resolve these situations on your own; your supervisor, having worked in the setting for much longer, will be in a better position to judge how best to handle the situation.

> How we feel about a situation is closely linked to how we appraise what has just happened. Before reacting, consider other possible appraisals; if necessary, seek input from others as to how they appraised the situation. If you are still upset, seek advice from your supervisor.

CONCLUSION

A wise adage is to "believe nothing of what you hear and only half of what you see." While this may sound an amusing comment, it is in fact grounded in the psychological paradigm that, ultimately, there is no reality, only perception. How you perceive, interpret, and respond to stimuli in your environment often says a lot more about you than the situation unfolding at hand. Always remember that there are often more than two sides to every story, and therefore, be willing to reappraise, to seek extra guidance, and to accept that, in the face of further evidence, your beliefs may be wrong. Awareness of and learning to overcome these common human errors of judgement will put you in a strong position to succeed in the challenging environment of modern medicine. Succeeding in the workplace as a professional uses all the skills of clear thinking outlined in this chapter. We will end with one final piece of advice: *Sometimes the best way to "think clearly" is to not always automatically believe what you think!*

LEARNING ACTIVITIES

1. Raise your awareness about your explanatory style by taking this short personal quiz. On a scale of 1 to 4, how much do you agree with the following statements? (1 = *not at all*; 4 = *very much so*)
   a. If I fail a test, I am certain it's my fault.
   b. Most people are inherently good.
   c. It's hard to really trust most people, because you never know what their real agenda is.
   d. I can easily overcome most of life's setbacks and obstacles.
   e. The world is becoming a more dangerous place.
   f. I feel confident about my future and the future of humankind in general.
   If you agreed more closely with the odd-numbered statements, your explanatory style tends to be more pessimistic; if you agreed more closely with the even-numbered statements, your style is more optimistic. If your answers were mainly in the middle, your style is somewhere between the two on the continuum.

2. In three or four sentences, describe a stressful situation that you have been in, and how you reacted. Write a paragraph on how your explanatory style as assessed in this chapter is likely to have affected your attributions and appraisals. Can you articulate how your explanatory style might explain part of your reaction to this situation? In retrospect, what could you have done better to improve the functional outcome of this situation?

3. Consider and discuss these scenarios with your classmates:
   a. Imagine two people are pointing your way at a shopping centre and laughing. You check your hair and make sure you haven't spilled anything silly on yourself but can find nothing wrong. What next? Do you still assume they are laughing at

you? At this point, what other reappraisals of this situation can you generate? Perhaps, they were laughing at something behind you or in your vicinity. Perhaps, one was gesturing as part of telling a joke and not pointing at you at all. Even if they *were* laughing at you, perhaps, it was for reasons not as sinister as you think—maybe you have a picture on your T-shirt that reminds them of a situation they were in together that was hysterically funny. See how many reappraisals you can generate. Write down the different emotional responses and reactions each causes.

b. An older adult patient makes a complaint against you of "mistreatment" during a recent attack of angina. He claims you were unnecessarily rough and demanding in ordering him to take his emergency medication and while taking his blood pressure. From the patient's point of view, what attributions and appraisals may have lead to this complaint? How could you respond to this complaint in a functional manner?

c. A doctor directs you to perform a procedure of which you have no knowledge or experience. Generate a few different appraisals to explain why the doctor has requested you to do this. With reference to your list of appraisals, what are some functional ways to respond to this request?

REFERENCES

Dutton, D. G., & Aron, A. P. (1974). Some evidence for heightened sexual attraction under conditions of high anxiety. *Journal of Personality and Social Psychology, 30*(4), 510–517.

Dykema, J., Bergbower, K., & Peterson, C. (1995). Pessimistic explanatory style, stress and illness. *Journal of Social and Clinical Psychology, 14*(4), 357–371.

Jackson, B., Sellers, R. M., & Peterson, C. (2002). Pessimistic explanatory style moderates the effect of stress on physical illness. *Personality and Individual Differences, 32*(3), 567–573.

Keinan, G. (1987). Decision making under stress: Scanning of alternatives under controllable and uncontrollable conditions. *Journal of Personality and Social Psychology, 52*(3), 639–644.

Lazarus, R. S. (1983). The costs and benefits of denial. In S. Bresznitz (Ed.), *The denial of stress* (pp. 1-32). New York, NY: Oxford University Press.

Martin-Krumm, C. P., Sarrazin, P. G., Peterson, C., & Famose, J.-P. (2003). Explanatory style and resilience after sports failure. *Personality and Individual Differences, 35*(7), 1685-1695.

Peterson, C. (2000). The future of optimism. *American Psychologist, 55*(1), 45-55.

Peterson, C., Seligman, M. E. P., & Vaillant, G. E. (1988). Pessimistic explanatory style is a risk factor for physical illness: A thirty-five year longitudinal study. *Journal of Personality and Social Psychology, 55*(1), 23-27.

Pham, M. T. (2007). Emotion and rationality: A critical review and interpretation of empirical evidence. *Review of General Psychology, 11*(2), 155-178.

Rule, B. G., & Nesdale, A. R. (1976). Emotional arousal and aggressive behaviour. *Psychological Bulletin, 83*(5), 851-863.

Seo, M.-G., & Barrett, L. F. (2007). Being emotional during decision making: Good or bad? An empirical investigation. *Academy of Management Journal, 54*(4), 923-940.

Taylor, S. E., & Brown, J. D. (1988). Illusion and well being: A social psychological perspective on mental health. *Psychological Bulletin, 103*(2), 193-210.

Tennen, H., & Affleck, G. (1987). The costs and benefits of optimistic explanations and dispositional optimism. *Journal of Personality, 55*(2), 377-393.

White, G. L., Fishbein, S., & Rutsein, J. (1981). Passionate love and the misattribution of arousal. *Journal of Personality and Social Psychology, 41*(1), 56-62.

Wild, J., Clark, E. M., Ehlers, A., & McManus, F. (2006). Perception of arousal in social anxiety: Effects of false feedback during a social interaction. *Journal of Behavior Therapy and Experimental Psychiatry, 39*(2), 102-116.

(6)   Being Convincing: Talking to Others Persuasively

Natoshia M. Askelson,
Mary Lober Aquilino, and
Shelly Campo

INTRODUCTION

As a new graduate, you will face numerous challenges. At the heart of many of these challenges is communication. This chapter will help you anticipate and prepare for the challenges you will face as you start your career and throughout the time you spend working in the health care environment. You will find skills and strategies to recognise potential challenges and handle them by communicating effectively and professionally. We will focus on helping you identify communication challenges both before and after they happen and showing you how to be proactive in solving these challenges.

THE STORY

I graduated five months ago from a basic nursing program. As a staff nurse in a paediatric haematology and oncology unit in a large teaching hospital, I was working one evening when I received a written order for pain medication for one of my patients. My immediate thought was that the order was the wrong dosage for the patient's weight. I looked up the drug information and talked with several of the more experienced nurses to verify my suspicion. I paged the resident, because I knew that the child needed the medication right away. After three pages and more than

75

an hour later, the resident called the unit. He was quite irritated that I had repeatedly paged him and questioned his order. I was frustrated because not only I was given an incorrect order, but also I was dealing with a young patient in pain and parents who were very distressed and upset with me for not helping their child immediately. The resident became curt, and I responded by becoming quiet. Although he did change the dosage, he did not acknowledge his error or my part in alerting him. I felt embarrassed, angry, and intimidated. After the phone conversation with the resident, the nurses whom I had consulted were not sympathetic. As a new nurse, I frequently question my own judgment and lack confidence in my ability. I look for multiple sources of validation before questioning medical orders. I am uncertain of the best way to question an order without appearing to challenge the doctor's knowledge and authority. I want to know more about how to approach someone with my ideas and persuade someone like this resident that I am right, without provoking anger. How do I communicate effectively to get the support I need and have the ability to handle challenges?

EFFECTIVE COMMUNICATION

Expectations and Understanding Your Audience's Behaviour

Communication challenges for nurses often involve being persuasive, particularly with colleagues you feel you need to convince to your point of view, with clients who may be reluctant to follow treatment advice, and in resolving disagreements with supervisors or medical officers. The most persuasive people have good communication skills. That is, they are good at listening, good at checking to make sure they understand, and then good at articulating their beliefs. Good communicators guide communication where they want it to go to meet their needs (Donohue & Kolt, 1992). Two key components in communicating effectively are to leave your biases (your expectations) at the door and to know your audience (understand why the person you are communicating with behaves as they do).

> Two key actions in beginning effective communications with others: (a) put your biases aside and (b) know who it is you are about to communicate with.

Probably the most important lesson you can learn as you start out in your career is the benefit of checking your own expectations at the door. What does that mean? Well, many communication challenges happen because we think things are going to be one way and they turn out another, or we *expect* people to behave one way and they behave differently. Our interpretation of situations and our reactions to them are explained by the expectancy violation theory (Burgoon & Hale, 1988). The violations of our expectations cannot only confuse us, but these violations can make us angry. For instance, if a nurse—like the one in our story—walks into a new job and expects coworkers like the resident to appreciate her pointing out of their mistakes, there will be several communication challenges. The nurse in our story also expected the resident to admit the mistake made and acknowledge the nurse's role in spotting the mistake. Obviously, this did not happen. Our nurse also expected to be thanked for using her skills to identify the wrong dosage. The nurse was very disappointed and upset because her expectations for her coworker's behaviour were not met.

Expectancy violation theory attempts to explain how we react to others' unanticipated behaviour (Afifi & Metts, 1998; Burgoon & Hale, 1988; Campo, Cameron, Brossard, & Frazer, 2004). When someone does something, we decide whether the behaviour violates our expectations. If it does, then we evaluate whether this violation is positive or negative. Did they behave better or worse than we expected them to? We also consider the degree of the violation. Was the person's behaviour radically different from that expected? If someone positively violates our expectations—that is, they do something that is unexpected, but that we view as "good"—we are likely to reward them. However, if someone negatively violates our expectations—that is, they do something unexpected that we view as "bad"—then we are likely to react negatively.

> Expectancy violation theory suggests that we need to make sure that we are aware of our expectations and how we react when people or situations do not match our expectations.

So, it's important that we understand our expectations, but it's also important that we understand people's behaviour. People have many reasons for their behaviour. Some reasons why people behave the way they do might be obvious, whereas others are not. Before stepping into a situation, people must consider why others behave the way they do. Attribution theory tries to explain how people make sense of other people's behaviour, or how people determine why others do the things they do (Heider, 1958). Broadly, the theory suggests that people attribute others' behaviour to internal attributes and external attributes (Weiner, 1986). The nurse in our story could have attributed the resident's behaviour to internal attributes (lack of sleep, horrible disposition) or external attributes (stressed because of the workload). Perhaps the nurse then judged the resident to be rude and egotistical and explained that this was why the resident did not acknowledge the nurse's ability to spot the mistake. She was then disappointed by how little her coworkers supported her and how little acknowledgment she received from all of her colleagues. Maybe she explained to herself that her coworkers were not helpful because they are mean and spiteful people. However, there could be other explanations. Perhaps the culture in that health care setting is not conducive to nurses supporting each other. Struggling through a new situation and learning the ropes might be considered a "rite of passage" in this setting and, by helping the less experienced nurses, the more experienced nurses would be robbing them of an important accomplishment. Perhaps, also, the resident was reluctant to admit the mistake because the resident is also new and unsure. Perhaps the resident didn't believe it was important to acknowledge the nurse's help because it was just expected that the nurse would spot these mistakes as part of the job of a competent nurse. Or perhaps the resident felt embarrassed and, not knowing the nurse well, did not feel safe in admitting his error. He might also have felt the desire to "save face" (we discuss face later in the chapter).

> Attribution theory suggests that we need to pay attention to possible internal and external factors that explain a person's behaviour and be careful not to draw false conclusions.

Most of us are guilty of overestimating the role internal factors such as personality and internal motivations plays in determining someone's behaviour (Nisbett & Ross, 1980), and we need to pay more attention to those external factors that might be important.

The Importance of Effective Communication for Health Care Professionals

Health care professionals must have effective communication skills. Effective communication decreases the number of negative patient outcomes (Anthony & Preuss, 2002; Coeling & Cukr, 2000) and increases employee morale (Smith, 2005). Like what we saw in the example of our new graduate, she had not been able to convince the resident that the dosage of the pain medication was wrong, which there might have been serious health consequences. Furthermore, if this nurse does not learn to communicate more effectively, she will become increasingly frustrated with her job. Effective communication is the foundation of good working relationships.

Health care professionals who do not develop effective communication skills tend to avoid communication that might lead to disagreement and do not have the ability to be persuasive. Such individuals are at risk for "groupthink." Groupthink occurs when people are unwilling to disagree or to voice concern, either of which can lead to negative consequences (Janis, 1982).

> Groupthink is a mode of thinking that people engage in when they are deeply involved in a cohesive in-group, when striving for unanimity overrides the concern to realistically appraise alternative courses of action. To avoid the trap of groupthink, don't be afraid to suggest other ideas or to disagree—respectfully!

In a health care setting in which people are not effective at disagreeing or raising concerns, medical errors occur and patients are at risk for negative health outcomes. Furthermore, effective communication will increase trust between health care professionals (Northouse & Northouse, 1997). After a discussion, both parties should have learned something about the other party and have a deeper understanding of where each other is coming from.

The Challenges of Communicating in the Health Care Setting

Communication challenges happen between people within a context and an environment. Communication can only be understood if the context and the roles people play are also understood. Specific components of health care settings can make communication tricky: power relationships, fast-paced environments, being overworked or stressed, lack of understanding about each other's roles, and different types of training can all interfere with communication.

The health care environment is a special place for communication. Communication issues frequently happen between nurses and physicians during the planning, implementing, and monitoring of patient care (Smith, 2005). Nurse–physician communication is often characterised by power difference between the two positions. There are unique power structures in health care settings, and power differentials are important for understanding communication in this arena (Northouse & Northouse, 1997). Power differentials can be made worse by the lack of understanding between the professions about who is responsible for which tasks and who has power over which decisions. Some power structures are explicit, like who outranks whom on the organisational chart, but other power structures might be related to who has access to certain knowledge or resources. In the story about our nurse, the resident held more explicit power, but the nurse's coworkers might have held power, in that they understood the culture of the workplace or had access to information that the new nurse needed. Understanding power relationships is important for understanding how to communicate effectively.

Health care professionals may also lack basic information about each other and each other's roles. Physicians do not know much about nursing education and what the day-to-day responsibilities and tasks of a particular nursing position are. Without this interprofessional understanding (Laschinger & Weston, 1995; Northouse & Northouse, 1997), it is hard to have appropriate expectations and effective communication. Nurses and physicians not only learn different skills, but their communication training is also different. Typically, nurses are trained to provide narratives that are descriptive and provide context, whereas physicians have been trained to communicate in a more action-oriented and decisive manner (Smith, 2005). These differences in communication styles alone can lead to challenges.

The health care setting is also fast paced. Decisions might have to be made quickly, either to save someone's life in an emergency or because there is little time to ponder or debate different solutions in a busy clinical setting. Medical care is complicated and, often, health care providers are juggling multiple patients with multiple health concerns. The fast-paced nature of the health care setting means that communication happens quickly, with little time to think about how to best formulate a message and with no time to explain a message that has been misunderstood.

To compound the issue, being overworked, lacking sleep, or working long hours make communication even more difficult. Health care providers not only have stressful jobs, but they also often experience role overload (Northouse & Northouse, 1997), which means that they are responsible for and do more than should be expected. All of these factors compound the issues around communication. Effective communication is hard when you are struggling to just get your job done!

With so much going on all at once in such a fast manner, sometimes in life and death situations, we should not be surprised that communication can break down. There is not a lot of time to consider how best to explain something vital in an emergency setting to someone who has more power than you do. Keep all of these challenges in mind while you read the following section on ways to be a better communicator and to be persuasive.

Key Strategies for Becoming a Good Communicator

A communicator must first strive to **understand where the other person is coming from** and why they act the way they do or hold the views they do. Only after understanding the audience will the communicator be able to make himself or herself understand and convey a persuasive message (Heider, 1958; Northouse & Northouse, 1997). Was the resident in our story dealing with another medical emergency? Were the nurse's coworkers threatened by the new nurse who held higher academic credentials?

Listening and being open are as important as talking. Part of striving to understand the audience is to listen to what people say and to pay attention to their emotions (Becze, 2009). The communicator needs to listen without interrupting. One way for people to check understanding and to demonstrate active listening is to summarise what has been heard and repeat it back to the audience. Additionally, all options need to be explored, including the opinions of those who were not previously concerned. Asking other parties for their ideas is vital.

Some power structures are unchangeable in the health care setting, but subtle, strategic and purposeful moves can alter power. There are two ways to increase the power of a person in a relationship: Either a person can increase the other person's dependence on them or they can decrease their own dependence on the other person (Donohue & Kolt, 1992). By taking on tasks or responsibilities that make others dependent on the nurse in our story, she could increase her power. She could also find ways to decrease her need for her coworkers. Perhaps she can find out key pieces of information in another way or use other sources to validate her concerns. The use of rewards can also increase a person's power. Rewards are something a person with power gives out, such as compliments, small favours, or other desirable actions. A person who gives out rewards appears more powerful. Perhaps the nurse could express her appreciation for the greater experience of her coworkers with different credentials.

A communicator needs to be credible to have an impact (Apker, Propp, Ford, & Hofmeister, 2006; Perloff, 1993). Credibility is about whether someone believes what is said. Credibility is also related to power. If one person's credibility is increased in another person's eyes, then the first person's power is increased in the relationship (Donohue & Kolt, 1992). People can convey credibility and increase the chances that someone believes them and trusts their opinion if they learn some key communication techniques. Good communicators avoid using jargon or terminology that is unnecessary and not precise. The use of big words does not necessarily make a communicator credible either. Communication must be tailored to the audience. A person's tasks, personality, and the context should dictate the communication style and content. Talking assertively and confronting conflict head on is the key to credibility. However, you must be assertive respectfully. The nurse in our story needs to build credibility with physicians and other nurses. This credibility will give her the ability to talk with authority and have people listen.

A large part of persuasion and finding solutions to communication challenges is dealing with people's face needs. Face is related to people wanting to be seen in a positive light (Wilson & Putnam, 1990). Being conscious of the face needs of the people you are working with is important. Face needs are going to be different for different people in different situations with various audiences (Wilson & Putnam, 1990). Face needs must be considered when preparing for effective communication and when seeking solutions to communication challenges.

There are four types of face needs. *Face maintenance* is related to one's good image. People with a good image are less likely to be attacked. If we are trying to convince someone to do something, we need to make sure that we have been maintaining our face, so someone else is more likely to believe us or be willing to comply with our requests. *Face saving* is what has to be done when something could potentially weaken someone's image. Face saving is a way to defend image. *Face attacking* is about making others look bad, so that we look good. This strategy is not recommended to get people to comply, but you need to be aware so that your actions are not interpreted as face attacking. *Face supporting* is about doing things that make someone else look good and increase the value of his or her face. The nurse in our story should play close attention to how she informs residents that they have made mistakes. Residents are likely to be highly motivated to save face and any questioning of their abilities could be seen as an attack.

Compassion and empathy are part of effective communication. To communicate effectively, a speaker needs to show consideration and pay attention to others' concerns (Apker, Propp, Ford, & Hofmeister, 2006). Empathy is about developing a new frame of reference (Northouse & Northouse, 1997) to understand an issue. Related to empathy is "culturally appropriate" communication for the health care setting (Arford, 2005). As we have outlined previously, the health care setting is a very special setting with a unique culture. Communication in this setting must be tailored to the culture. For most health care settings, this means that the communication needs to be brief and organised in a way that is useful to the receiver and based on evidence or fact. If the communicator expects either an action to be taken or a direct response, this expectation also needs to be communicated. In the health care setting, there is not enough time to completely explain each other's worldviews (Arford, 2005). Thinking about the nurse in our story, how should she use compassion and empathy? She needs to remember to be culturally appropriate in her communication with the resident. Perhaps she needs to learn more about how nurses question physicians' orders in her setting, or to acknowledge that perhaps, the resident was having a difficult day.

An effective communicator in the health care setting is assertive (Smith, 2005). Being assertive does not mean that the communicator is a bully or aggressive; instead, the communicator speaks concisely and authoritatively when trying to communicate a message. Here are some tips for becoming a more assertive communicator (Smith, 2005):

- Attract the person's attention. There are many ways to attract a person's attention: use his or her name, so he or she knows someone is talking to him or her; make eye contact; and be face-to-face. When people are distracted, they are harder to persuade (Petty & Brock, 1981).
- State the concern in a clear and succinct way.
- State the problem that is causing the concern. Use a clear, strong voice to state the problem. If the speaker rambles or speaks too softly, the point either will be lost or will not seem important.
- Have a solution ready. If the speaker brings a solution to the table, the conversation will move in the direction of a resolution.
- Go to the final step to reach an agreement with the other person— more about getting to this point later in this chapter.

When our nurse communicated with the resident, she needed to make sure that the resident was listening by asking for his full attention, telling him that she was unclear about the dosage in the order and that she believed it to be wrong and stating what she believed the correct dosage to be.

Communicators have to control their emotional responses. Using emotion to handle a difficult situation will make it harder. Determining the cause of an emotional response to understand how to control the response may be helpful (Pettrey, 2003). The nurse in our story was certainly stressed while trying to reach the resident as she struggled to provide comfort to a patient in pain and handle concerned parents. To not become emotional when she finally was able to speak with the resident may have been very difficult. Learning to keep a check on emotional responses takes practice and time.

Three tips to keep emotions in check when stressed:

1. Write down what you think is upsetting you.
2. Calm and center yourself with three deep breaths held for the count of 5. The key is to feel the breath in your chest or abdomen by putting all of your attention there. Think the words "relax," "calm," and "focus."
3. Write down the next course of action.

The communicator should identify similarities or commonalities between themselves and the audience (Cialdini, 2001; Pettrey, 2003). Identifying and communicating these shared needs and interests help develop a sense of homophily, meaning that the other person recognises the ways in which the communicator and he or she are similar. Persuading someone is easier if you can make him or her see how similar you are or that you have similar goals. Focus on similarities rather than differences. Perhaps the resident and the nurse have been working the same night or weekend shifts for a while. Pointing out how tiresome the shift has become or how both of them are missing an important event in their community because they are at work might help develop some homophily between the two health care providers.

Selecting solutions that benefit both parties will make persuasion easier (Pettrey, 2003). People who see some advantages for themselves in a proposed change are easier to convince than those who can see no benefits for themselves.

A neutral setting is best for these conversations (Becze, 2009). However, finding such a place might not be easy in the health care setting. At the very least, try to avoid settings in which patients, family and friends of patients, or other noninterested parties can overhear or become involved.

Nonverbal communication should not be ignored. People often forget that we communicate in ways other than words (Northouse & Northouse, 1997). Our facial expressions, our hands, or the way we stand or sit all communicate something using body language. Body language should match verbal communication. Standing with your arms crossed does not signal that you are open for compromise. We are more conscious of some body language than others are. We may be able to control eye rolling and huffing, but how we sit and what we do with our arms while talking are harder to control; we have to be more conscious of that kind of body language.

Addressing communication challenges requires courage and commitment (Pettrey, 2003). Many people find it easier to ignore issues or to keep their concerns to themselves. This type of behaviour can hurt patients and make life less content for the person who decides not to address communication issues. Being willing to attack a communication challenge head on is no easy matter. Being an effective communicator and persuading people is an ongoing process that requires vigilance and the commitment to always improve your communication and persuasive skills. If the nurse in our story continues to feel bad about not having her skills acknowledged, she will not have the resilience needed to stay happy in her profession.

Persuasion is an important element of effective communication. Persuasion means convincing other people to do something or to change their minds and should happen without coercion or force—people should willingly change their minds or adopt new behaviours. There are many evidence-based strategies for persuading people; we have outlined a few here:

- One strategy is called *foot-in-the-door* (Burger, 1999; Freedman & Fraser, 1966). This strategy gets its name from the idea that we ask someone to do a small task or make a small change and we have our foot in the "door" of his or her mind. Once the foot is in that door, we are able to ask him or her for more extensive changes or behaviours. The strategy is based on the idea that most people consider themselves as someone who gets along with others and who can easily accommodate others. Because of this basic assumption, people are more likely to comply with a small request first and then with a subsequent bigger request.
- The *door-in-the-face* strategy is again based on the idea that people like to think of themselves as willing to help others out (Cialdini, Cacioppo, Bassett, & Miller, 1978; O'Keefe & Hale, 1998). For door-in-the-face, the first request is something that is outrageous or more than what one would expect from a normal person. When the request is turned down because it is outrageous, the person who said "no" feels a bit guilty about turning it down. The requester then turns around and asks for a more reasonable request. The other person is then more likely to comply with this second more reasonable request because he or she feels guilty for not helping the first time and wants to maintain a helpful self-image. Furthermore, in comparison to the first outrageous request, the second request appears easy or simple.
- *Positive reinforcement* is based on the work of B. F. Skinner (1974). This strategy involves rewarding people for the behaviours you want them to perform. The reward increases the chances of their repeating the behaviour in the future. The key to this strategy is figuring out what constitutes a positive reward for the person you are trying to influence. Although a verbal compliment in front of peers or superiors might be enough for some people, other people might expect bigger,

more tangible rewards such as willingness to take on an extra patient, work a shift in an emergency, or do some extra paperwork.

- *Reciprocity* is a strategy (Cialdini, 2001) that people use every day. In layperson's terms, we are referring to "give and take" or "you scratch my back, I'll scratch yours." If you do a favour for someone, he or she is inclined to want to pay you back. By making people feel more indebted to you, you might be able to exercise more influence over them and persuade them to do what you would like.

- *Attitude-behaviour consistency* suggests it is easier to persuade someone to do something if you point out to him or her that his or her attitudes and behaviours are not consistent. This strategy draws heavily on the idea that people are uncomfortable with holding attitudes that are different from their behaviours, and they feel that they must change one or the other (Festinger, 1957). For instance, if someone is usually very excited about the latest technological gadget, but refuses to consider adopting the most up-to-date clinical guidelines, pointing out this inconsistency maybe helpful (Snyder & Kendzierski, 1982).

CONCLUSION

Communication is a large part of the workday for health care professionals. At times, you might feel overwhelmed, so here are a few key points to remember:

- Each party shares some responsibility for creating the communication challenge and for solving it (Pettrey, 2003).
- We have control over some things and other things we do not have control over. Changing people is impossible, but their behaviour or how you react to them can be changed.
- Although it is sometimes hard to believe, most people do not behave the way they do because they are evil or are out to make your life hard. This is why we suggest that you be aware of your expectations or biases before you go into a situation. Your predictions about someone's internal motivations are not likely to be the most important determinants of his or her behaviour. People usually see their own behaviour as rational and making a lot of sense. In addition, they probably don't realise how their behaviour affects others.

■ Because communication challenges can become overwhelming and some people find that they expend energy and emotion worrying about these kinds of situations, keeping these challenges in perspective is important:

  ■ This challenge is only a small part of your life (Pettrey, 2003).
  ■ Action can make the situation better (Pettrey, 2003).
  ■ This challenge is not personal and should not negatively affect relationships (Pettrey, 2003).
  ■ A person cannot spend all his or her time and energy focused on one challenge (Pettrey, 2003). Be sure to know when you need to walk away for a while.

Whether a communication challenge has been handled successfully or not so successfully, reflect and determine what lessons you can learn from it. By learning from past mistakes and successes, you are ensuring growth in your ability to communicate effectively. Effective communication begins with identifying your expectations and realising how they may not be in line with reality. Then, think critically about why the people in your work environment behave the way they do.

LEARNING ACTIVITIES

1. *Role-play.* Find a partner. You and your partner are going to role-play the story we described at the beginning of this chapter. One of you can be the nurse, while the other plays the resident. Try to use the techniques and strategies outlined in this chapter to make this story have a better ending. What were the nurse's expectations going into the conversation? How does the nurse start the conversation after the resident has called back? How does he or she works towards more a productive outcome?

2. Search the Internet for "tips for keeping emotions in check." Identify at least three more strategies to assist this nurse (and perhaps yourself in the future) to ease the natural tendency to become emotional when faced with a communication challenge.

3. Recall the concept of "groupthink" raised in this chapter. Construct a verbal response to the scenario that follows that would help to avoid the occurrence of groupthink but would also enable the participants to save face and feel respected.

Scenario: You are receiving a morning handover. A senior nurse discusses a patient, Mr. Smith, someone you have come to know from previous admissions. He has developed a chronic, hospital-acquired wound infection and is feeling depressed at his ongoing ill health. The senior nurse states, "Not much we can do for this patient. He's a case for the social workers."

REFERENCES

Afifi, W. A., & Metts, S. (1998). Characteristics and consequences of expectation violations in close relationships. *Journal of Social and Personal Relationships, 15*(3), 365-392.

Anthony, M. K., & Preuss, G. (2002). Models of care: The influence of nurse communication on patient safety. *Nursing Economics, 20*(6), 209-215.

Apker, J., Propp, K. M., Ford, W. S. Z., & Hofmeister, N. (2006). Collaboration, credibility, compassion, and coordination: Professional nurse communication skill sets in health care team interactions. *Journal of Professional Nursing, 22*(3), 180-189.

Arford, P. H. (2005). Nurse–physician communication: An organizational accountability. *Nursing Economics, 23*(2), 72-77.

Becze, E. (2009). Deal effectively with conflict in the workplace. *ONS Connect, 24*(2), 26.

Burger, J. M. (1999). The foot-in-the-door compliance procedure: A multiple-process analysis and review. *Personality and Social Psychology Review, 3*(4), 303-325.

Burgoon, J. K., & Hale, J. L. (1988). Nonverbal expectancy violations: Model elaboration and application to immediacy behaviours. *Communication Monographs, 55*(1), 58-79.

Campo, S., Cameron, K. A., Brossard, D., & Frazer. M. S. (2004). Social norms and expectancy violation theories: Assessing the effectiveness of health communication campaigns. *Communication Monographs, 71*(4), 448-470.

Cialdini, R. B. (2001). *Influence: Science and practice* (4th ed.). Boston, MA: Allyn and Bacon.

Cialdini, R. B., Cacioppo, J. T., Bassett, R., & Miller, J. A. (1978). Low-ball procedure for producing compliance: Commitment then cost. *Journal of Personality and Social Psychology, 36*(5), 463-476.

Coeling, H. V. E., & Cukr, P. L. (2000). Communication styles that promote perceptions of collaboration, quality, and nurse satisfaction. *Journal of Nursing Care Quality, 14*(2), 63-74.

Donohue, W. A. & Kolt, R. (1992). *Managing interpersonal conflict.* Newbury Park, CA: Sage Publications.

Festinger, L. (1957). *A theory of cognitive dissonance.* Stanford, CA: Stanford University Press.

Freedman, J., & Fraser, S. (1966). Compliance without pressure: The foot-in-the-door technique. *Journal of Personality and Social Psychology, 4*(2), 195–202.

Heider, F. (1958). *The psychology of interpersonal relations.* New York, NY: John Wiley & Sons.

Janis, I. L. (1982). *Groupthink: Psychological studies of policy decisions and fiascos* (2nd ed.). Boston, MA: Houghton Mifflin.

Laschinger, H. K. S., & Weston, W. (1995). Role perceptions of freshman and senior nursing and medical students and attitudes toward collaborative decision making. *Journal of Professional Nursing, 11*(2), 119–128.

Nisbett, R. E., & Ross, L. (1980). *Human inference: Strategies and shortcomings of social judgment.* Englewood Cliffs, NJ: Prentice-Hall.

Northouse, P. G., & Northouse, L. J.. (1997). *Health communication: Strategies for health professionals* (3rd ed.). Standford, CT: Prentice Hall.

O'Keefe, D. J., & Hale, S. L. (1998). The door-in-the-face influence strategy: A random-effects meta-analytic review. *Communication Yearbook, 21,* 1–33.

Perloff, R. M. (1993).*The dynamics of persuasion.* Hillsdale, NJ: Lawrence Erlbaum Associates.

Pettrey, L. (2003, February). Who let the dogs out? Managing conflict with courage and skill. *Critical Care Nurse, AACN Critical Care Careers Supplement,* pp. 21–24.

Petty, R. E., & Brock, T. C. (1981). Thought disruption and persuasion: Assessing the validity of attitude change experiments. In R. E. Petty, T. M. Ostrom, & T. C. Brock (Eds.), *Cognitive responses in persuasion* (pp. 55–79). Hillsdale, NJ: Lawrence Erlbaum Associates.

Skinner, B. F. (1974). *About behaviourism.* Toronto, Canada: Random House.

Smith, I. J. (2005). *The joint commission guide to improving staff communication.* USA: Joint Commission on Accreditation of Healthcare Organizations.

Snyder, M., & Kendzierski, D. (1982). Acting on one's attitudes: Procedures for linking attitude and behaviour. *Journal of Experimental Social Psychology, 18*(2), 165–183.

Weiner, B. (1986). *An attributional theory of motivation and emotion.* New York, NY: Springer-Verlag.

Wilson, S. R., & Putnam, L. L. (1990). Interaction goals in negotiation. In J. A. Anderson (Ed.), *Communication yearbook 13* (pp. 374–406). Newbury Park, CA: Sage Publications.

(7) Mind Games at Work: Preparing for Effective Team-Working

Tony Warne and Sue McAndrew

INTRODUCTION

The philosopher Epictetus wrote that man is disturbed not by things but by the view he takes of them. This idea is the key to our discussion about learning to become more resilient when working as part of a team. Much contemporary health care relies on teamwork, whether it be interprofessional (such as nurses working with fellow nurses) or multidisciplinary (such as when teams of different professions work collaboratively). Although teams have been described as providing a "protective veneer to the stress of work" (Edwards, 2005, p. 142), they also sometimes become a quagmire for intrapersonal and interpersonal conflicts. The focus for this chapter is the self in relation to others. In this context, an understanding of the games often played out in interpersonal encounters (in this instance, multidisciplinary teams) is useful. Understanding can emphasise the need for you to develop resilience strategies that enable conflict to change into collaboration. The chapter introduces the reader to the concept of developing a personal store of "resilience." Self-esteem and self-efficacy form the basis of this store of resilience, because both are interrelated parts of how we think of our self in relation to others and how others can influence this sense of self. An example of the complexity of such processes is illustrated in the following story. The story is drawn from our experience of many hours spent in such meetings. Although the content is entirely fictitious, the story is based on real people we have worked with. Woven into the story are the communication and metacommunication of the various participants as they experience different aspects of the meeting. These communications and metacommunications are shown as italics.

THE STORY: AT WARD ROUND

Dr. White enters the ward at 9.43 a.m. Looking into the office, he informs the ward manager that whenever they are ready, the ward round can begin. The ward manager immediately leaves the office with Dr. White and goes to the meeting room, informing other members of staff of the impending meeting as she goes. Slowly, the other members of staff invited others to enter the room *(Ward manager: Do they not realise Dr. White is waiting?)*. Sitting quietly, the participants wait for the meeting to start. Dr. White is engrossed in conversation with the ward manager and does not appear to notice that everyone is now ready for the meeting to begin *(Staff nurse: Typical of them making us wait)*. Perhaps, sensing a change in atmosphere, Dr. White looks up, coughs, and comments how pleasing it is to see the full team in attendance.

Opening a set of case notes, Dr. White reads for a few minutes before starting to discuss the first patient—Mary—and her impending discharge. After stating that Mary appears to have made good progress and could be discharged within the next 2 days, Dr. White invites the ward manager to comment *(Dr. White: We need to discharge Mary, but I can't remember where we are up to with her—the ward manager will come to my rescue)*. After briefly listening to what the ward manager has to say, Dr. White turns and then asks "the team" if anyone else has further comment, or should they ask Mary to come in and tell her of the decision *(Staff nurse: Mary's not really ready for discharge but there is no point in saying anything because they have already made up their minds to get rid of her)*. A student nurse leaves the room to find Mary and bring her into the meeting. Mary is invited to sit down opposite to Dr. White, between the new registrar and the community nurse, neither of whom she has previously met *(Student nurse: Poor Mary, she looks really scared, but no one will listen to me pointing this out)*. Dr. White informs Mary that she will be discharged the following day, and that the community nurse (sitting next to her) will call and see her in a week's time *(Community nurse: I wish Dr. White wouldn't do that. This is the first time I've seen Mary and she looks as worried as me. I wonder what she will expect of me)*.

Dr. White, then, asks if Mary would like to say anything *(Student nurse: I think Mary is going to cry. I feel uncomfortable for her—I couldn't say anything in front of these people)*. Mary becomes upset and checks that Dr. White is aware of the circumstances, which are still at home, that led to her suicide attempt *(All staff look down, feeling very uncomfortable, but no one feels able to speak up)*. At this point, the social worker makes comment about the stressful environment Mary has been living in but hesitates and then stops as no one else appears to be listening *(Social worker: I just feel embarrassed now. Is it worth trying to speak up for patients when no one is in the least bit interested in what I have to say? They just have no time for social workers)*. Dr. White looks at the clock and then informs Mary that the team believes that she is better now and more able to cope with the problems at home *(Mary: Dr. White is very busy, but I wish someone would just listen to me. Perhaps I don't deserve being listened to; perhaps other people are far worse off than me)*. Mary sobs into her handkerchief as the ward manager nods to the student nurse to take Mary out of the room *(Ward manager: I wish some of the team would speak up a bit more. There is only so much I can say and do)*. Dr. White picks up the next set of case notes and starts to read. *(Dr. White: I like the idea of teamwork, but it's difficult at times to keep up with what responsibilities each of these other professionals have . . . it's sometimes hard to get a clear picture of who is doing what . . . the boundaries seem blurred, indistinct)*.

PLAYING TEAM GAMES

Some argue that effective multiprofessional teamwork is linked to positive patient outcomes, job satisfaction, team morale, and staff retention (Stein-Parbury, 2007; Thomson, 2007). However, the preceding story makes clear that intrapersonal and interpersonal dynamics can compromise the effectiveness of teams by the way these dynamics are played out.

In 1967, Stein provided an illustration of how these intrapersonal and interpersonal dynamics play out in the way doctors and nurses communicate with each other when trying to ensure good patient care. He called these ideas the "doctor–nurse game" (Stein, 1967). His ideas reflected the wider societal attitudes and values prominent at the time, particularly those around gender, social position, and power. For example, in this game, Stein argued that nurses should only make suggestions for patient care in a manner that ensures the suggestion appeared to be initiated by the doctor rather than the nurse. Consider our scenario and how the ward manager rescued Dr. White. Stein suggested that if the game was played correctly, the resulting doctor–nurse relationship would be mutually beneficial. If the game was played incorrectly, then it would lead to many difficulties for the doctors, nurses, and patients. By following the correct rules of the game, nurses and doctors can prevent open conflict, albeit adopting this approach is also likely to hinder effective communication.

Stein (1967) also claimed that the so-called subservience of the nurse and dominance of the doctor in this relationship was a charade. He claimed that nurses were often deeply involved in decision making. In playing the game, nurses were enabled to inform and advise the doctor without appearing to challenge the doctor's position or authority. In Stein's doctor–nurse game, the doctor, by tradition, was held to have total responsibility for decisions about patient management. Paradoxically, however, in order for doctors to make the best decisions possible for "their" patients, the doctors require access to a wide range of comprehensive information. Nurses' input constitutes an important source for this information. Unfortunately, although nurses' input is considered valuable, this input is not recognised, acknowledged, or respected. So, in playing the game, nurses remain largely invisible (Deacon, Warne, & McAndrew, 2006).

Today, Stein's work around the doctor–nurse game has been challenged because of the lack of evidence underpinning his theory. The doctor–nurse game idea does, however, serve to illustrate that harnessing the benefits of teamwork, collaboration, and partnerships can be difficult to achieve. For example, although games have a repetitive quality, when one is part of the game, distinguishing and making sense of the game can be difficult. Likewise, aspects of power, influence, competition, and politics, both within and between individuals, professions, and professionals, need to be recognised and openly addressed (Warne & Stark, 2004). Openly addressing these team behaviours and dynamics can provide a new way for individuals to learn about themselves and others. However, to achieve this, we believe that effective team-working is better *caught* rather than *taught*.

One way of catching effective team-working is to use experiential learning. However, in this approach, the opportunity for team members to learn to effectively read the story, the experience or the situation is sometimes missing. We believe that to gain insight into how others are influencing our sense of self, learning must involve a "layered" reading of such stories. We illustrate this method by returning to our preceding story and, in reappraising the situation, adopt a layered presentation of what might be going on.

The Outer Layer

For many of us, and particularly as newly qualified practitioners, often the first (and sometimes only) reading of a situation is largely superficial and descriptive. For example, in our story, we could describe the scenario as simply a multiprofessional team in operation. Clearly, this level is a starting point only and is largely inadequate—what we describe as the surface encounter. What lies under this surface may not always be easily visible. Consider an initial reading of the effectiveness of the team in our scenario.

On the surface, you might think it is effective. The meeting starts on time. Both the consultant and the ward manager are present and other members of the team join them. Case notes are produced and read, and some discussion is invited. A decision is made and the patient is told of the team's decision. Although the patient becomes a little upset, the doctor is reassuring and the patient is given discharge. The team seems effective. During this process, the doctor invites other members of the team to contribute to the discussion, and the team appears to work well as the discussion is kept to a minimum and actions are taken. No one appears to want to strongly contest any of the decisions taken, perhaps indicating that the team members are happy to support each other. So perhaps, is this a collegial team?

Exposing the Second Layer

However, what these surface impressions do not allow is access to the interpersonal dynamics of the various relationships in play here. Many teams find that the way in which the team is set up and the chosen way of working together results in tensions being experienced by individual team members. When these tensions are not properly addressed, poor team relationships, de-motivated team members, ineffective communication and the nonachievement of team objectives can result (Warne & Stark, 2004). The metacommunication (in italics in our story) shows the different and divergent perceptions that reveal the often hidden professional rivalries and power struggles.

Being aware, understanding, and making sense of these different perceptions of reality can be difficult. In the context of team-working, students may well be taught concepts of good team-working such as "effective communication," "shared values," and "respect for other professionals." However, simply being aware of such concepts is unlikely to help the student understand what is going on in this meeting or to understand how these interactions affect the self and, subsequently, the response to others. In such situations, self-esteem and self-efficacy are challenged. The individual in a new or unfamiliar situation is at risk of having both compromised. The response is often a movement from accepting the presence of risk to the more defensive position of passive adaptation to protect one's self-esteem and self-efficacy. In reality, such a position is likely to provide protection. However, personal security is achieved only through recourse to rules, procedures, and established processes. Intuition and experience are abandoned, resulting in decreased confidence in one's own sense of self (Warne & McAndrew, 2010).

Layer Three: Splitting

Experiencing a reduced sense of self-efficacy can also give rise to further tensions. The perceptions of what conceptually constitutes effective team-working can often sit side by side with power relations, status, resource limitations (organisational and self), blurred role definitions, and time pressures. All of these factors can affect the team dynamics. In dealing with such inconsistencies and tensions, nurses often resort to the defence mechanism of "splitting." Splitting, in this instance, is not dividing into "good" and "bad" but rather into the lesser of two evils: blaming organisational problems, lack of resources, hierarchical positions, loss of trust in oneself and others, loss of self-worth, or the insecurity of not knowing. For example, in our story, the community nurse may have been left thinking: *Typical of Dr. White . . . no introductions, no getting to know the patient, just expects to discharge whomever to free up precious beds. And we can go in and deal with all the problems still facing the patient when she returns home to the same situation that got her into hospital in the first place. And if that isn't bad enough, I will have to discharge someone else from my caseload in order to accommodate Dr. S's latest command. Obviously, the work I do is not that important.*

This example reveals that, perhaps at one level, resources are blamed for the community nurse's perception of the negative outcomes of the meeting. However, at the same time, self-doubt and mistrust is evident. The community nurse, at the second layer, was starting to doubt her professional and personal self, but this doubt is then projected onto Dr. White's professionalism, leadership, and team membership. In projecting blame onto Dr. White or organisational resources (beds), the community nurse is, to a certain degree, able to negate her own mistrust of self and self in relation to others. Just as in Stein's game, this use of an unconscious defence mechanism helps reduce the inner conflict and compromised sense of self. The benefits are, however, only short term. Games prevent honest, intimate, and open relationships between players. Instead, to improve self-esteem and self-efficacy (and thus, develop and maintain a resilience store), a person needs to bring the psychodynamic processes involved in communicating to conscious awareness. For the community nurse, this would offer the opportunity to share her own feelings and concerns with the team, who would hopefully reaffirm her value as a team member. In this way, her self-doubts and mistrust are not left to fester in her unconscious.

We argue that nurses also need to learn how to deconstruct group interactions (Warne & McAndrew, 2009) in ways that don't reduce their thinking to simply categorising team members as *good* and *bad* or teams as *effective* and *ineffective*. Rather, the approach must reveal the interpersonal dynamics of multiprofessional teams. Such an approach enables synergy of the theory and practice of team-working. The first step in this process is understanding who we are in terms of our own self-worth and self-efficacy. Initially, positive early parent–child relationships and external support systems that encourage and reinforce coping efforts (Rutter, 1987) are vital to developing a healthy sense of self. However, concepts of self are not static from childhood but continue to be modified by life experiences. For example, the everyday situation of the multiprofessional meeting provides a context in which self-identities are established, changed, and maintained. Processes of negotiation enable us both to "define the situation" in which we find ourselves and to "construct a reality."

Knowing Me and My Part

The concept of self can be understood as a belief that a person holds about himself or herself as a person and as a person who is interacting with others in the world (Epstein, 1973). The sense of self forms the basis of our resilience store. Two aspects are particularly important in this regard: self-esteem and self-efficacy. Self-esteem is the dimension of individual difference that captures the individual's feeling of his or her own value. Self-efficacy refers to an individual's belief in his or her ability to control events in his or her life, particularly those events that have significance for him or her. For nurses, both these aspects are subject to constant challenge as their sense of personal and professional self-interactions with what can often be diametrically opposing organisational exigencies and demands. We suggest that a well-established feeling of one's own worth as a person, together with a confidence and conviction that one can cope successfully with life's challenges, will provide resilience when confronted with such demands.

However, the difficulty of constructing and maintaining a positive sense of self is increased by the component of self in relationships with others. Critically, personal relationships are fundamental to effective team-working (Gelso, 2002), and other people are often part of achieving one's goals. As we can tell from the preceding story, such interactions are often ends in themselves. For example, in our story, these ends include monitoring the impact of treatment, discharging the patient, and so on. Because of these interdependencies on others, people both shape and are shaped by their social interactions. Relationships are thus influenced by both the personalities of and communications with those engaged in team-working (Gelso, 2002). An individual's sense of self provides the framework that guides the interpretation of his or her social experiences and regulates his or her participation in these experiences. This process can be seen in situations in which the roles of individuals are *taken* and *given*, as in our multiprofessional team meeting. Consider the impact on the social worker (in the role of Mary's advocate) of not being listened to, or the impact on the student nurse of being indirectly told to get on and deal with a distressed Mary. As Goffman (1959) noted in his most famous work, *The Presentation of Self in Everyday Life*, we are at once both the outcomes and creators of these encounters. People learn about themselves from others, both through social comparisons and through direct interactions and, in this respect, social comparison can be a potent source of self-knowledge, self-esteem, and self-efficacy (Schoeneman, 1981).

Developing a Resilience Store

As discussed in other chapters of this book, resilience is sometimes thought of as the ability we have to positively adapt to and rebound from significant adversity and the resultant distress (Everly, Welzant, & Jacobson, 2008; McAllister & McKinnon, 2009). Much of the research undertaken on resilience has explored the individual's ability to recover from traumatic events. However, in this chapter, we have conceptualised a resilience store as reserves that can be drawn on to deal with what are often the stressful experiences of team- working.

We argue that the turbulent and somewhat messy realities of working as part of a health care team should be embraced and not seen as something to avoid. New ways of working, shifting values, changing politics, and partnerships will constantly emerge, and preparing nurses in dealing with these diverse issues is vital. Foster, McAllister, and O'Brien (2006) noted the relationship between some personal qualities and the abilities of nurses. A well-developed self-awareness, an acceptance of self and others' feelings, an understanding of the complexity of the human experience, and an ability to accept ambiguity and uncertainty were positively related to performance. Nurses draw on these qualities and abilities in constructing therapeutic relationships with their patients. We argue that nurses need to be better prepared to recognise and use these personal qualities and abilities to achieve the best outcomes for themselves and others.

> A resilience store could include well-developed self-awareness, an acceptance of self and others' feelings, an understanding of the complexity of the human experience, and an ability to accept ambiguity and uncertainty.

Returning to the layering of our scenario, the way in which the game was played out obviously gave rise to tensions for many team members. Inherent tensions exist in all relationships between independent identities with different agendas. We need to recognise and accept that real differences in intergroup relations are part of our humanity. Likewise, viewing the conflict phase of group development (the storming phase) as a transformational process involving change and growth can be useful (Tuckman, 1965). Small steps can contribute to changes in intragroup dynamics and can lower the intensity of group conflict (Rothman, 1992). Drawing from your own resilience store helps clarify what you need to retain a separate identity whilst supporting others. Changes often come with the rehumanising of those we previously blamed for our angst. This change in our own attitude facilitates relationship building that stimulates creative, rational compromise and also affects the more primal choices between trust and mistrust, hatred and friendship (Gopin, 2002).

In creating and maintaining a resilience store, we need to recognise that the very things that first enabled us to build our store are the things we continue to need throughout life. We can obtain these things from others if we are also prepared to offer them to others: promoting social support, nurturing friendships, seeking role models, being open-minded and flexible in the way we think about problems, and avoiding rigid and dogmatic thinking; all help to achieve mutual respect, responsiveness, and inner trust within each other. In such an environment, change can be accommodated as the group metamorphoses (Winnicott, 1965). During this phase, power differentials can be challenged and relationships redefined. However, change can only occur from within; you can change yourself, but you cannot change others or how yourself is viewed or experienced by others. All parties have to accept responsibility for change if teamwork is to be successful.

CONCLUSION

Contemporary health care relies on teamwork and in this chapter, we have explored, through the use of a layered scenario, how nurses can be better prepared to work in this way. The focus for this chapter has been on self in relation to others and how an understanding of the games often played out in multiprofessional teams can better prepare people to develop resilience strategies that enable conflict to be changed into collaboration. The layered deconstruction of the relationships inherent in team-working highlights the complexities and dilemmas involved in developing a self-concept. Nurses can use this technique to develop, maintain, and access what we refer to as a resilience store. Self-esteem and self-efficacy form the basis of the resilience store, both being interrelated parts of how we think of our self in relation to others, and how others influence this sense of self. The ability to consciously access your resilience store, particularly in times of conflict, provides opportunities to nurture supportive relationships, seek positive role models, be open minded, and develop empathy for others. In doing so, you will gain mutual respect, responsiveness, and inner trust that will foster more collaborative ways of working.

LEARNING ACTIVITIES

Discuss the following points in groups with your classmates. Then bring your insights to a whole-of-class discussion.

1. In an ideal health care system, organisational structures are usually put in place to facilitate more effective multiprofessional team-working. Often, these structures bring together health and social care resources (money and people) and aim to blur previous organisational boundaries. What problems could arise in trying to agree approaches that ensure the best possible care is provided by different agencies and professionals?

2. In the doctor–nurse game, nurses were to be totally subservient to the doctor. According to Stein (1967):

> The cardinal rule of the game is that open disagreement between the players must be avoided at all costs. The nurse can communicate her recommendations without appearing to make a recommendation statement. The physician, in requesting a recommendation from a nurse, must do so without appearing to be asking for it. (p. 482)

> Think about a team you have been involved with or observed. Who held the power in that team? Why did they hold the power—what behaviours did they display and how and what did they communicate to maintain their position of power? What did other members of the team do to reinforce that power?

3. Make a list of what is in your own resilience store. Now, make a list of people in a team that you work with. Of the people you have listed, identify those you feel are your friends and those who might be considered "foe." Now, return to your resilience store and think about the attributes that you have listed. Consider how you could use these attributes to positively improve your interpersonal relationships with those whom you find difficult to engage.

REFERENCES

Deacon, M., Warne, T., & McAndrew, S. (2006). Closeness, chaos, and crisis: The attractions of working in acute mental health care. *Journal of Psychiatric and Mental Health Nursing, 13*(6), 750-757.

Edwards, K. (2005). The phenomenon of resilience in crisis care mental health clinicians. *International Journal of Mental Health Nursing, 14*(2), 142-148.

Epstein, S. (1973). The self-concept revisited or a theory of a theory. *American Psychologist, 28*(5), 404-416.

Everly, G., Welzant, V., Jacobson, J. (2008). Resistance and resilience: The final frontier in traumatic stress management. *International Journal of Emergency Mental Health, 10*(4), 1-10.

Foster, K., McAllister, M., & O'Brien, L. (2006). Extending the boundaries: Auto-ethnography as an emergent method in mental health nursing research. *International Journal of Mental Health Nursing, 15*(1), 44-53.

Gelso, C. (2002). Real relationship: The something more of psychotherapy. *Journal of Contemporary Psychotherapy, 32*(1), 32-40.

Goffman, E. (1959). *The presentation of self in everyday life.* New York, NY: Doubleday.

Gopin, M. (2002). Religion, violence, and conflict resolution. *Peace and Change, 22*(1), 1-31.

McAllister, M., & McKinnon, J. (2009). The importance of teaching and learning resilience in the health disciplines: A critical review of the literature. *Nurse Education Today, 29*(4), 371-379.

Rothman, J. (1992). *From confrontation to cooperation: Resolving ethnic and regional conflict.* London, England: Sage Publications.

Rutter, M. (1987). Psychosocial resilience and protective mechanisms. *American Journal of Orthopsychiatry, 57*(3), 316-331.

Schoeneman, T. (1981). Reports of the sources of self-knowledge. *Journal of Personality, 49*(3), 284-294.

Stein, L. I. (1967). The doctor-nurse game. *Archives in General Psychiatry, 16*(6), 699-703.

Stein-Parbury, J. (2007). Understanding collaboration between nurses and physicians as knowledge at work. *American Journal of Critical Care Nursing, 16*(5), 470-478.

Thomson, S., (2007). Nurse-physician collaboration: A comparison of the attitudes of nurses and physicians in the medical-surgical patient care setting. *Medical Surgical Nursing, 16*(2), 87-93.

Tuckman, B. (1965). Developmental sequence in small groups. *Psychological Bullitin, 63*(6), 384-399.

Warne, T., & McAndrew, S. (2009). Constructing a bricolage of nursing research, education and practice. *Nurse Education Today, 29*(8), 855-858.

Warne, T., & McAndrew, S. (2010). Mirror, mirror: Reflections on developing the emotionally intelligent practitioner. *Mental Health and Learning Disabilities Research and Practice, 6*(2), 157-169.

Warne, T., & Stark, S. (2004). Service users, metaphors and team working in mental health. *Journal of Psychiatric and Mental Health Nursing, 11*(6), 654-661.

Winnicott, D. W. (1965). *The maturational processes and the facilitating environment.* Madison, CT: International Universities Press.

(8) Thriving in the Workplace: Learning From Innovative Practices

Debra Jackson, Glenda McDonald, and Lesley Wilkes

INTRODUCTION

Nurses need to thrive in workplaces that are often challenging and even personally harmful (Jackson, 2008a; Jackson, Clare, & Mannix, 2002; Jackson & Daly, 2004). These issues are extensively documented in the literature and have been related to the reasons for nonretention of nurses in the workplace (Jackson, Mannix, & Daly, 2003; Stordeur, D'Hoore, & the NEXT-Study Group, 2006). In order to establish a successful career, nurses need to learn to manage these elements of the workplace environment and develop personal strategies that are meaningful to them as practitioners of their own resilience. This chapter focuses on the importance of resilience in dealing with workplace adversity. Professional support networks are presented as one innovative strategy that can be applied to help support the development of resilience in nurses and midwives experiencing workplace adversity. In the following story, Kylie, a new nursing graduate, reminds us of some of the inherent potential challenges of the nursing work place.

KYLIE'S STORY

I look out of the kitchen window into the quiet night sky. Thank goodness, that shift is over . . . I feel so exhausted. I'm relieving the way things are at work—snapped words, raised eyebrows, the continuous hurried

105

pressure, and the sense of being on eggshells . . . the sense that one wrong word or step could spell disaster. It's like a film playing over and over in my head. I don't feel comfortable there, or confident about what they think of me. They don't trust me and I don't know them. I would like to be able to ask for help, but no one has any time and then he or she will just think I am incompetent, anyway.

I don't have any family or close friends and my partner works shifts as well. They are so short staffed at work—I never know when I'll be asked to work an extra shift, or whom I'll be working with. I just can't take it if I find out I'm working with some of them, I feel so stressed—I would rather just work on my own. I feel I'm not productive . . . not living up to expectations, and I worry that I'll get into trouble.

When I was at the unit, I had the clinical facilitator, plus the other students, to talk to if there were any problems, and we always debriefed back on campus. I miss that camaraderie and would really like to have someone to debrief with and just talk things over with. I could talk to someone at work, but I don't know anyone well enough and I don't want it to get around and everyone to think I can't hack it. I really want to find some ways of improving my working life.

WHAT IS WORKPLACE ADVERSITY?

Workplace adversity is the term given to describe aspects of the working environment or organisation that are experienced by workers as difficult, unhelpful, or potentially harmful to their safety and wellbeing (Jackson, Firtko, & Edenborough, 2007). Health care workplaces are recognised as having the potential to be challenging, difficult, and even capable of producing harmful effects on staff. Numerous sources of workplace adversity have been identified in the literature, including excessive workloads, shortages of staff, lack of support, interpersonal difficulties, abusive work environments, shift work, feeling devalued and uncared for. and organisational change and restructuring (Gabrielle, Jackson, & Mannix, 2008; Hutchinson, Vickers, Jackson, & Wilkes, 2006; Speedy, 2004).

> Be aware of the concept of "workplace adversity"—harmful conditions facing workers that can lead to dissatisfaction, exhaustion, and burnout.

The demands of the health environment require that nurses and midwives consider how workplace adversity may affect them and the quality of care that can be provided to clients or patients in such an environment. The literature suggests that workplace adversity may affect the ability of nurses and midwives to work effectively and to achieve autonomy and job satisfaction. Additionally, the degree to which professional nonjudgmental and inclusive collegial relationships can be established has been questioned (Jackson, 2008a; Rotenberg et al., 2008). If workplace adversity is ignored, staff members may not care for themselves adequately. Thus, the daily challenges faced by nurses and other health practitioners can eventually lead to emotional exhaustion and may result in burnout (Vallido, Jackson, & O'Brien, 2009). The challenge is to develop healthy workplaces that foster collaboration and support between nurses.

Working in Large Organisations

Workplace adversity can create problems for the nursing workforce that health care organisations may not be well equipped to handle. Most delivery of health services occurs within the context of very large organisations. Even though some health organisations are small and are seen as more friendly and cohesive, workplace adversity can still exist. Health care organisations are in an almost constant state of flux. They operate under pressure because there is nearly always a high demand for service, and this, coupled with a continual shortage of resources, creates particularly challenging working environments.

The concept of organisations being unreasonable and hurtful to employees is not new. Both Fromm (1942/1960, 1963/1994) and Blauner (1964) described organisations as alienating places and highlighted the possibility of employees experiencing feelings of fragmentation, meaninglessness, isolation, and powerlessness. The very nature of nursing means that, in some ways, nurses are particularly vulnerable to the negative effects of work in large organisations. Factors such as variability of working hours, role stress, and poor sleep quality—all of significance for nurses—have been found to negatively influence worker's health and wellbeing (Camerino et al., 2008; Costa, Sartori, & Akerstedt, 2006; Lambert et al., 2004).

WHAT IS RESILIENCE?

Resilience is defined as the capacity of individuals to withstand significant change, adversity or risk and is enhanced by protective factors within individuals and environments (Jackson et al., 2007). Researchers have used the concept to understand why some people react to adversity in ways that result in a loss of function whereas others continue to function effectively, even in the face of major difficulties.

The protective characteristics of resilience have been discussed in Chapter 1. Jackson et al. (2007) identified several characteristics of resilience in the workplace context: "building positive and nurturing professional relationships; maintaining positivity; developing emotional insight; achieving life balance and spirituality; and becoming more reflective" (p. 1). As suggested earlier in this chapter, the many sources of workplace adversity in current health care environments can potentially affect the health and wellbeing of nurses and other health workers. However, there are strategies that may be used to counter these negative elements. The development of personal resilience can play a part in helping nurses and midwives make the ever-present and challenging decisions about their own self-care and self-development. Furthermore, increasing personal resilience can help nurses and midwives navigate their professional and personal lives and better cope with the challenges of working within a large and pressured organisation.

> Resilience is a key strategy to empower your practice and to protect you from workplace adversity. Resilience can be fostered by being positive, surrounding yourself with like-minded colleagues, having work-life balance, and learning from experiences through reflection.

PROFESSIONAL SUPPORT NETWORKS

In the vignette we presented at the beginning of the chapter, graduate nurse Kylie identifies a lack of support and the desire to confide in a trusted professional friend about how she is managing in the workplace. Her story reveals a sense of loneliness and isolation that is quite overwhelming.

Clearly, some sort of support is needed for Kylie. However, she has not disclosed this need to those in the workplace who could help her, and she seems to be at risk of withdrawing from potential workplace support.

Collegial support and constructive collegial relationships have been identified as essential to affirmative and positive work environments and to the ability of nurses and midwives to thrive in the workplace (Jackson, 2008b). Kylie's story reveals that she does not feel she can talk to anyone about her feelings. Her narrative betrays a sense that any discussion of her feelings could be construed as weakness, or an inability to cope with the challenges of life as a working nurse. Yet, the failure to share her feelings means that people may not realise how vulnerable she is feeling, and so may not reach out to offer support and encouragement. A very old saying tells us that a problem shared is a problem halved, and some quite considerable relief can be had through the act of sharing experiences and stories with interested and supportive peers, many of whom may have had some similar experiences. However, as Kylie's narrative reveals, people do not always feel safe to disclose these types of difficulties.

A key strategy that could provide almost immediate support for Kylie and help to transform her experience of working as a nurse would be to develop a professional support network. A professional support network describes a set of helpful connections with key people that Kylie can use for help and support as needed. The network can comprise a mix of more senior or more experienced people and peers who may be having similar experiences. The professional network can be drawn from people both within and external to the current workplace. For example, graduate nurses in other wards or hospitals can be valuable sources of support and may be able to provide helpful advice and counsel. So educators and other clinical experts in the health setting and people involved in professional organisations can represent excellent sources of support, too.

A crucial element of such network could be the identification of a suitable mentor. Mentoring is becoming more common in nursing and midwifery in Australia and internationally (Jackson, 2008c; McCloughen, O'Brien, & Jackson, 2006, 2009).

Mentoring

Notwithstanding the fact that there are many acceptable definitions (McCloughen et al., 2006), effective mentoring relationships have several common characteristics. These characteristics include trustworthiness, mutual respect, accessibility, and holding shared understandings about the nature and aim of the relationship (McCloughen et al., 2006).

Although the concept of mentoring has been widely recognised and applied in business for generations, recognition has come somewhat more recently to nursing and midwifery (McCloughen et al., 2006). However, since that time, nurses have embraced the concept with formal mentoring programs being offered in a wide range of clinical and hospital settings (Grindel & Hagerstrom, 2009; McVeigh, Ford, O'Donnell, Rushby, & Squance, 2009; Mills, Francis, & Bonner, 2008). Some programs have drawn on more senior nurses to mentor younger or less experienced colleagues, with the added benefit of retaining older nurses and midwives. Mentoring also effectively develops positive relationships between generations of nurses and midwives who may have differing work values and perspectives (Leners, Wilson, Connor, & Fenton, 2006; Sherman, 2006; Wieck, 2007).

Independently, starting up your own mentoring relationship—without a formal program—is also possible and may be more successful than those relationships that are formalised in and mediated through prescribed channels in the workplace (Jackson, 2008c). Jackson (2008c) describes professional generosity in the nursing workplace and suggests that helpful and supportive relationships, though not always identified as mentoring in a formal sense, actually have many of the qualities of mentoring.

> A key strategy for you and your colleagues: Access or initiate a mentoring program. Contact your professional nursing association to find out if there is a program available for your region.

LESSONS LEARNED: THE VALUE OF PROFESSIONAL SUPPORT

Therefore, what are the lessons we can learn from Kylie's story? Kylie commenced her career as a registered nurse and, simultaneously, the support strategies at the university—she had found useful and to which she had become accustomed, were lost to her. This combination of circumstances meant that, in a relatively short time, she experienced negative emotions about her work. We need to remember that entering the graduate workforce represents a major change. Though graduation marks the beginning of life as a registered nurse or midwife, it also initiates a significant change of lifestyle. Simultaneously, loss of the supportive network of university academic staff and support people occurs, as well as the loss of the day-to-day support and camaraderie of fellow students. These changes can make graduates vulnerable to workplace adversity, and so they need to take measures to develop personal resilience.

Developing "positive and nurturing professional relationships" (Jackson et al., 2007, p. 1) has been identified as an important characteristic of personal resilience. One of the ways to develop these positive and nurturing relationships is through creating a professional support network. Obviously, a personal network will change and grow over time as new workplace connections are forged, but it is advantageous to identify a professional network early on, before entering a new environment.

CONCLUSION

The many potential sources of professional support in health care workplaces, in addition to the personal support networks comprised of family and friends, have a vital role to play in developing and maintaining resilience and in promoting positive feelings of wellbeing in challenging workplaces.

LEARNING ACTIVITIES

1. Discuss the following questions in small groups with your classmates: Can you identify the types of workplace adversity being experienced by Kylie? What strategies could Kylie draw on to help her deal with the situation? Have you experienced any similar feelings when working in the clinical environment? What strategies did you draw on to help? What other strategies would you use in future?

2. Think about these questions and then discuss your thoughts with the class: How would you go about establishing a professional

support network? What qualities would you look for in a mentor? What would you want from a mentoring relationship? In addition to a mentor, what other sorts of people and relationships would you seek in forming a professional support network?

3. Write down or create a computer file identifying the key people you would seek in forming your own professional support network.

4. Search the Internet to find some award-winning employers and compare and contrast their characteristics. These websites may get you started:

http://www.employmentspot.com/top-lists/100-best-hospitals-to-work-for/

http://www.greatplacetowork.com.au/best/list-bestusa.htm

REFERENCES

Blauner, R. (1964). *Alienation and freedom: The factory worker and his industry.* Chicago, IL: University of Chicago Press.

Camerino, D., Conway, P. M., van der Heijden, B. I., Estryn-Be'har, M., Costa, G., & Hasselhorn, H. M. (2008). Age-dependent relationships between work ability, thinking of quitting the job, and actual leaving among Italian nurses: A longitudinal study. *International Journal of Nursing Studies, 45*(11), 1645–1659.

Costa, G., Sartori, S., & Akerstedt, T. (2006). Influence of flexibility and variability of working hours on health and well-being. *Chronobiology International, 23*(6), 1125–1137.

Fromm, E. (1960). *Fear of freedom.* London, England: Routledge and Kegan Paul Ltd. (Original work published 1942)

Fromm, E. (1994). Alienation. In H. Clark, J. Chandler, & J. Barry (Eds.). *Organisation and identities: Text and readings in organisational behaviour* (pp. 391–396). London, England: Chapman and Hall. (Original work published 1963)

Gabrielle, S., Jackson, D., & Mannix, J. (2008). Adjusting to personal and organisational change: Views and experiences of female nurses aged 40–60 years. *Collegian, 15*(3), 85–91.

Grindel, C. G., & Hagerstrom, G. (2009). Nurses nurturing nurses: Outcomes and lessons learned. *MEDSURG Nursing, 18*(3), 183–194.

Hutchinson, M., Vickers, M. H., Jackson, D., & Wilkes, L. (2006). Workplace bullying in nursing: Towards a more critical organisational perspective. *Nursing Inquiry, 13*(2), 118-126.

Jackson, D. (2008a). Servant leadership in nursing: A framework for developing sustainable research capacity in nursing. *Collegian, 15*(1), 27-33.

Jackson, D. (2008b). Collegial trust: Crucial to safe and harmonious workplaces. *Journal of Clinical Nursing, 17*(12), 1541-1542.

Jackson, D. (2008c). Random acts of guidance: Personal reflections on professional generosity. *Journal of Clinical Nursing, 17*(20), 2669-2670.

Jackson, D., Clare, J., & Mannix, D. (2002). Who would want to be a nurse? Violence in the workplace—a factor in recruitment and retention. *Journal of Nursing Management, 10*(1), 13-20.

Jackson, D., & Daly, J. (2004). Current challenges and issues facing nursing in Australia. *Nursing Science Quarterly, 17*(4), 352-355.

Jackson, D., Firtko, A., & Edenborough, M. (2007). Personal resilience as a strategy for surviving and thriving in the face of workplace adversity: A literature review. *Journal of Advanced Nursing, 60*(1), 1-9.

Jackson, D., Mannix, J., & Daly, J. (2003). Nursing staff shortages: Issues in Australian nursing homes. *Australian Journal of Advanced Nursing, 21*(1), 44-47.

Lambert, V. A., Lambert, C. E., Itano, J., Inouye, J., Kim, S., Kuniviktikul, W., . . . Ito, M. (2004). Cross-cultural comparison of workplace stressors, ways of coping and demographic characteristics as predictors of physical and mental health among hospital nurses in Japan, Thailand, South Korea, and the USA (Hawaii). *International Journal of Nursing Studies, 41*(6), 671-684.

Leners, D., Wilson, V., Connor, P., & Fenton, J. (2006). Mentorship: Increasing retention probabilities. *Journal of Nursing Management, 14*(8), 652-654.

McCloughen, A., O'Brien, L., & Jackson, D. (2006). Positioning mentorship within Australian nursing contexts: A literature review. *Contemporary Nurse, 23*(1), 120-134.

McCloughen, A., O'Brien, L., & Jackson, D. (2009). Esteemed connection: Creating a mentoring relationship for nurse leadership. *Nursing Inquiry, 16*(4), 326-336.

McVeigh, H., Ford, K., O'Donnell, A., Rushby, C., & Squance, J. (2009). A framework for mentor support in community-based placements. *Nursing Standard, 23*(45), 35-41.

Mills, J., Francis, K., & Bonner, A. (2008). Walking with another: Rural nurses' experiences of mentoring. *Journal of Research in Nursing, 13*(1), 23-35.

Rotenberg, L., Portela, L. F, Banks, B., Griep, R. H., Fischer, F. M., & Landsbergis, P. (2008). A gender approach to work ability and its relationship to professional and domestic work of nursing personnel. *Applied Ergonomics, 39*(5), 646-652.

Sherman, R. (2006). Leading a multigenerational nursing workforce: Issues, challenges, and strategies. *Online Journal of Issues in Nursing, 11*(2), 13.

Speedy, S. (2004). Organisational violations: Implications for leadership. In J. Daly, S. Speedy, & D. Jackson (Eds.), *Nursing leadership* (pp. 145–163). Sydney, Australia: Churchill Livingstone.

Stordeur, S., D'Hoore, W., & the NEXT-Study Group. (2006). Organisational configuration of hospitals succeeding in attracting and retaining nurses. *Journal of Advanced Nursing, 57*(1), 45–58.

Vallido, T., Jackson, D., & O'Brien, L. (2009). The effective nurse. In R. Elder, K. Evans, & D. Nizette (Eds.), *Psychiatric and mental health nursing* (pp. 2–11). Melbourne, Australia: Elsevier.

Wieck, K. L. (2007). Motivating an intergenerational workforce: Scenarios for success. *Orthopaedic Nursing, 26*(6), 366–371.

What to Do When the Busy Day Is Over

Jane Brannan, Mary de Chesnay, and Patricia L. Hart

INTRODUCTION

The purpose of this chapter is to provide you with various ideas for relaxing and letting go of your tension from work. Although you may be familiar with these strategies, when you are actively experiencing stress from a high-pressure job—as a new graduate trying to acculturate to your practice setting, for example—you may forget to implement them. Ruminating about what happened that day at work and taking short cuts such as eating fast food and watching television, instead of a healthy meal and exercising, is all too easy. However, you must remember that your work is only *one* aspect of your life, all-consuming though it may seem at times. To be a success in nursing, you must be a success in life. The ideas in this chapter will help you to remember that life is much more than work. Taking time for some of the suggested activities, or others that you find fun, is essential to make sense of life when you work in a high-pressure job. In this chapter, we will present some examples of how you might react under stress and then discuss how you might react in a more self-affirming way. We also discuss coping strategies from the literature that are generally helpful in dealing with stress.

SARAH'S STORY

"FAST PACED AND PATIENT TURNOVER." This is the motto for the Short-Stay Unit where I work. Our patient population usually consists of patients who have surgical procedures performed and need to be monitored for 24 to 48 hours post-op. I graduated 3 months ago from nursing school. This story tells what happened to me not long ago, on my first day after orientation, when I was given my own patient assignment. My assignment included two thyroidectomy patients, two laparoscopic cholecystectomy patients, and a young man who had had an appendectomy. The night nurse reported that all my patients had an uneventful night. As I was getting started with my rounds, the call light went off in one of the thyroidectomy patient's rooms. He was complaining of difficulty in breathing. He was extremely restless and said that he could not get enough air. He had this funny sound as he breathed in . . . I guessed that he was having inspiratory stridor, but I had never heard this sound before in a real patient. I examined his thyroidectomy dressing site and noted a haematoma the size of a golf ball. My heart was pounding in my chest . . . what should I do? I needed to get help *now*! My hands were shaking so badly that I could barely grab the phone to activate the Rapid Response team. I raised the head of the bed and put on the oxygen cannula. Almost immediately, help from the unit arrived, as well as the Rapid Response team. I telephoned the surgeon and gave him the assessment information. The patient's respiratory status continued to deteriorate. The Rapid Response team leader called a code. The code response physician intubated the patient's airway with much difficulty. The surgeon arrived and the patient was whisked off to the operating room for emergency exploratory surgery and decompression of the haematoma. I then made a call to the patient's wife and told her of the incident and that her husband was now in the operating room having emergency surgery. She was hysterical on the phone and I had a difficult time really knowing what to tell her and how to comfort her. By this time, my knees were shaking so badly that I could barely stand and I felt like I was going to faint.

I'm not sure if I'm cut out to work on this type of unit. This patient could have died and I'm not sure if I want that responsibility on my hands. This was my first emergency situation and I wasn't sure what to do. I'm worried about the responsibility of caring for people and making wrong decisions that might affect their lives. I dread going to work now. I don't want to think about all this stuff, but I can't seem to stop. I just can't relax. I'm even dreaming about caring for patients and agonising over what decisions I should make.

COPING WITH STRESS IN NURSING

The preceding story presents some of the issues that we'll talk about in this chapter. Sarah is frustrated and fearful. Confidence typically wanes during the first 6 months after graduation (Casey, Fink, Krugman, & Propst, 2004), so finding ways to feel supported, comforted, and buoyant are essential when beginning your practice. In this chapter, we have included some strategies that nurses often use to balance their work and home life and cope with stresses they are experiencing. Included are strategies related to building supportive relationships, meditation, embracing your spiritual life, pet therapy, volunteering, and using music, humour, and exercise.

Responding effectively to health crises is one of the most challenging experiences for nurses. Learning how to *consciously apply* coping mechanisms is the key. Otherwise, you may find yourself simply reacting to, and thus vulnerable to, the pressures of nursing work.

Building Support Bridges

Building professional and nonprofessional relationships is vital in establishing a support system. Support systems provide you with different options for guidance and emotional support throughout your career.

Colleagues
You need to build positive, nurturing relationships with colleagues that provide a safe haven for letting off emotional steam. Connecting with colleagues gives you opportunities to relate, vent about stressful situations, and reaffirm that you are not alone in dealing with the trials and tribulations of your work environment. Just being able to talk to someone who "walks in your shoes" and who can relate to your situation helps you work through your stress and frustrations. Colleagues with more experience can provide you with guidance and insights into challenging situations and can explore positive solutions with you. Finding a trusted professional colleague with whom to share your experiences also provides a nurturing relationship for that person as well.

"Having a support person is very important. I work in a
pediatric cancer unit. Just dealing with the emotional
aspects of this type of work is very stressful. I am lucky
because I found a friend on the unit that I can confide in.
At the end of the day, I can call Susan and talk about
how the day went. She understands what I am going
through since she works on the same unit and experiences the same situations that I do. We have developed a
bond over the past year. I don't know what I would have
done as a new graduate nurse if I did not find someone
like Susan to lean on." (Pam, new graduate nurse)

You can build your professional support system by connecting with
social networks such as professional nursing organisations and nursing
listservs. The bottom line is finding a support system that works for you
and provides the right outlet that allows you to refill your emotional
bucket. Here is a list of nursing community websites that may be useful:

- Nurses and midwives: http://www.nursesandmidwives.com/
- Royal College of Nursing, Australia: http://www.rcna.org.au/
- AllNurses: http://allnurses.com
- CareNurse: http://www.care-nurse.com
- Nurse Connect: http://www.nurseconnect.com
- Nursing Link: http://nursinglink.monster.com
- Nurses Reconnected: http://www.nursesreconnected.com/

Family and Friends
You also need to develop support systems outside of your work environment. Being able to vent to a neutral person who does not have an invest-
ment in your work provides a "sounding board" for bouncing off ideas in
a nonthreatening manner. Support from family and friends helps validate
you and grounds you back into your personal values and beliefs. Connecting with family and friends provides you with a sense of belonging
and reaffirms your sense of self-worth. Just sitting with a friend, enjoying
a cup of coffee or hot chocolate, visiting with a family member, or attending a social event helps rejuvenate your emotional health. Just knowing
that you have your family and friends to lean on in times of stressful situations provides a "solid rock" to hang on to.

"I came from a big family who lived together on a farm in rural Virginia. As farmers, we relied on each other for everything—food, clothing, and shelter. I always felt crowded in the farm house having to share a room with my three brothers and I couldn't wait to move up to the city for nursing school. Then I took a job in the ICU and it wasn't very long before I realized just how important they were to me and how much I missed just being with them. I was really glad when texting was invented. Now, we email and text all the time." (Brad)

Meditation

You can use meditation as a way to increase calmness and physical relaxation, improve your psychological balance, or enhance your overall wellness. Meditation focuses your attention so you are mindful of your thoughts, feelings, and sensations and are able to observe them in a nonjudgmental way. Using meditation allows you to control the flow of your emotions and the thoughts in your mind, and helps you to focus and concentrate in your day-to-day activities. Meditation has several health benefits, such as reducing your blood pressure, relaxing your muscles, reducing anxiety, and eliminating stressful thoughts. Meditation also helps you learn to "stay in the moment" and connect with yourself, known as *centring*. Centring allows you to focus on the "here and now," and provides time to calmly rejuvenate your mind (U.S. Department of Health and Human Services, National Institutes of Health, & National Center for Complementary and Alternative Medicine, 2009).

Meditation does not have to be a "religious" activity. There are many styles of meditation, but all have the four common elements listed here (U.S. Department of Health and Human Services et al., 2009). So, find a quiet place and give meditation a try.

- **Select a quiet location.** Many meditators prefer a quiet place with as few distractions as possible, which can be particularly helpful for beginners. People who have been practicing meditation for a longer period sometimes develop the ability to meditate in public places, like waiting rooms or buses.

■ **Choose a specific and comfortable posture.** Depending on the type being practiced, meditation can be done while sitting, lying down, standing, walking, or in other specific positions.

■ **Focus your attention.** Focusing one's attention is usually a part of meditation. For example, the meditator may focus on a mantra (a specially chosen word or set of words), an object, or simply the rise and fall of the breath.

■ **Have an open attitude.** An open attitude during meditation means letting distractions come and go naturally without stopping to think about them. When distracting or wandering thoughts occur, they are not suppressed; instead, the meditator gently brings attention back to the focus. In some types of meditation, the meditator learns to observe the rising and falling of thoughts and emotions as they spontaneously occur.

Spirituality

Some nurses find support in their faith and spirituality. Spirituality is defined as a "basic or inherent quality in all humans that involves a belief in something greater than the self and a faith that positively affirms life" (Miller, 1995, p. 257). Spirituality provides a means to explore finding meaning and purpose in your life and how that meaning relates to yourself, family, and community. Finding purpose and meaning to your life leads to a sense of fulfilment. Nurses find that when they are more aware of their own spirituality, they are able to help and care for their patients and families in a more holistic way. Through spirituality, nurses are able to retain some balance in their life and put stressful situations into a perspective that allows them to move on (Ablett & Jones, 2007; Tugade & Fredrickson, 2004; Tusaie & Dyer, 2004).

"Working in a hospice facility is very difficult. I deal with terminally ill patients on a daily basis. I think if I did not have my faith and spirituality to fall back on, I wouldn't be able to renew myself each day to come back to work. I know there is a higher power that is looking over my shoulder and guiding me in caring for my patients. I pray each night to give me strength to care for my patients and help them deal with their end-of-life issues." (Nancy)

Pets as Healers

In the previous sections, we discussed building support systems such as making friends at work and using meditation to reduce your job stress. Now, we shift to other sources of comfort. A large body of literature supports the role of pets in promoting health and wellbeing (Garrity, Stallones, Marx, & Johnson, 1989; Kidd & Kidd, 1985; McNicholas & Collis, 2006; Wells, 2007). Although causal associations between companion animal ownership and the alleviation of symptoms of specific diseases have not been definitively shown (Wells, 2009), it is a widely held belief in Western culture that pets are a good source of social support and may, in fact, be healers in their own right. Ask any pet owner!

What can you do if you do not have a pet? What if you cannot have a pet because of housing restrictions or allergies? Although companion dogs and cats are the most common pets, many people enjoy the calming effect of watching fish in an aquarium or having a small caged pet such as a guinea pig. Simply interacting with your friends' pets can be restful. Offer to pet-sit when they are away, or simply make a point of holding and petting the animals when you visit your friends.

> "When I was a new graduate, I had an Airedale terrier who used to go everywhere with me that I was allowed to take him. I would have taken him to work if I could because he really earned the title of "best friend." I used to come home exhausted from the emergency room but no matter how tired I was, I knew I needed to take him for a walk and then feed him. And no matter how cranky I was, he always greeted me so enthusiastically as if I was the most wonderful person alive. We would walk and then go home and sit by the fire and I would tell him about my day. He would listen attentively for about 15 minutes and then suddenly yawn and I knew that was my signal to put it behind me." (Mary)

Volunteerism

Volunteer activities can reduce stress by helping to refocus one's attention from the problems and concerns at work to making a contribution to a worthy organisation. Many organisations like local animal shelters, shelters for sufferers of domestic violence, or church groups that feed the older adult are rarely sufficiently staffed or funded. Offer to help out your chosen organisation for a day, a week, a weekend, or a month. Some groups such as domestic violence shelters have training requirements. Others will take any help they can get, but prefer to have someone commit to a specific schedule.

An exciting opportunity for nursing students in many programs is to volunteer their services to poor communities, both in their own countries and abroad. The faculties that accompany them speak of the richness of the experience for volunteer nurses in the communities in which their students work (de Chesnay, 2005). Welch (2009) wrote about her extensive volunteer activities on medical missions to Central America in terms of how rewarding it was to spend time in a community and get to know the people. Even the smallest intervention can make a huge difference in people's lives.

> "I work in a high-pressure intensive care unit and when I come home from work, I am usually too tired to think of anything but sleep. But every Sunday morning, I train myself to go to church and teach a Sunday school class. Working with small children who are excited to hear the Bible stories I tell them is so energizing that I remember that there is more to life than people dying."
> (Kate, ICU nurse)

Music

"Take a music bath once or twice a week for a few seasons. You will find it is to the soul what a water bath is to the body" (Oliver Wendell Holmes [1809-1894], U.S. author and physician). Music has been a basic part of human life in every culture throughout history. During the Crimean War, Florence Nightingale was a proponent of careful consideration of all environmental needs of patients, including music to aid in healing. Music therapy has been provided for patients for many years and has been found to provide physical, as well as emotional benefits. The physical effects of music include lower blood pressure and heart rate, lower respiratory rates in ventilated patients, and overall patient satisfaction (Good et al., 2001; Nilsson, Rawal, & Unosson, 2003). In addition, Cooke, Holzhauser, Jones, Davis, and Finucane (2007) found that music, in combination with aromatherapy massage, significantly reduced anxiety in nurses in an emergency department.

Music is a mode of self-care that is very individual in terms of preference, but is a universal soother. After the busy day is over, music is a safe haven of self-care. As Maya Angelou (1974) describes, taking refuge in music can be a way of relieving stress. Playing, singing, or listening to music can provide respite from the stresses of the day. Some have described the feeling of playing music both as a physical sensation and creating an art piece. The detachment from other thoughts provides a mental resting time. Whether playing, singing, or listening, the use of music for relaxation and unwinding is an excellent option to cope with the stress of the day.

Humour and Laughter

You have heard the old cliché, "Laughter is the best medicine." Adding humour and laughter into your life has many benefits such as strengthening your immune system (Bennett, Zeller, Rosenberg, & McCann, 2003; Berk, Felten, Tan, Bittman, & Westengard, 2001), relieving stress and anxiety (Abel & Maxwell, 2002; Iwasaki, MacKay, & Mactavish, 2005), reducing pain and discomfort (Mahony, Burroughs, & Hieatt, 2001), and improving your quality of life (Svebak, Kristoffersen, & Aasarod, 2006). You may have had the opportunity to watch the movie, *Patch Adams*, which portrayed the life of Hunter "Patch" Adams, MD. Adams was one of the first medical practitioners to discuss the value of incorporating therapeutic humour and laughter into his bedside routine in caring for his patients.

You may experience or participate in black humour, sometimes referred to as aberrant or "gallows humour," during stressful or difficult situations in the workplace. The term *gallows humour* was first coined by Sigmund Freud in his theory of humour (Freud, 1905/1960). Freud believed that individuals use joking as a method to relieve anxiety and stress when dealing with feelings of pain, fear, and horror. As a word of caution, the use of gallows humour may seem inappropriate to others. What is funny to one group of health care providers may not be funny to another group (Bennett, 2003).

Begin to look for opportunities that bring humour and laughter into your life—watching funny movies, reading the funny pages, drawing pictures with young children, or going to a comedy club. The bottom line is to find mirthful activities that bring a smile to your face and laughter into your heart.

"Working in the busiest emergency room in the city has its stresses. You never know who or what is coming in the door. One minute the ER is quiet and the next minute chaos has erupted. Patients with gunshot wounds, traumatic injuries from auto accidents, heart attacks, and strokes are just a few types of cases I see every day. Some days, I don't even get to take a break or eat lunch. Working in this type of environment, I have learned to add humor and laughter into my life. It helps me relieve my stress and keeps me grounded in the simple things in life. I really like going to the comedy club after work on weekends. A group of us from the ER go and we just have the best time laughing and cutting up. I can tell that this stress outlet helps me to cope with the demands of working in the ER." (Robert)

Exercise to Energise

"Those who think they have not time for bodily exercise will sooner or later have to find time for illness" (Edward Stanley, Earl of Derby, 1873). Frequently, new graduates find stress relief by blogging their thoughts. The following is a blog from a new graduate (you can find many of these online by doing a Google search for "blogs by new nurses"):

OK . . . think! . . . get the blood cultures from the central line and log them in to the computer. Whose IV pump is beeping? Uh oh . . . That lady doesn't look like she did early this morning . . . maybe she needs some oxygen. Oh no! Her O2 sats are 88%. Do something! Now the sweet elderly man in 816 wants some tea for his wife. Just a minute, I'll be right there. There goes that IV alarm again! It's 10:30 already and I haven't even given meds. Think! What's next? It goes on and on . . . I'm just feeling so stupid today . . . like I don't know how to do anything . . . 1 pm and I am stressed. I swallow my sandwich in 10 minutes still wondering if I'll ever get finished today . . . and I glance outside at the sunshine. A quick walk in the sun, deep breathing, and stretching. It just took 20 minutes and it is amazing how much clearer my head is. What is it about just walking that does that to a person? Endorphins? Fresh air? The hospital has an inside walking track too—convenient. It's been the only a few weeks but I'm finding that a 20 or 30 minute walk right after work is what I crave to clear my head and ready myself for going home at the end of the day. And I feel so much better—like things aren't as bad as they were when I started walking. (Barbara Jean, new graduate, RN)

It's hard to imagine that anyone would suggest more exercise after an exhausting day of caring for patients. Isn't that *enough* exercise already? Not really. During each day, you've gone through enough activation of your stress response to completely deplete your body's physical resources via increased muscle tension, increased heart and respiratory rates and blood pressure, and chemical reactions brought on by the stresses of the job each day. Lazarus and Folkman (1984) found that long-term stress is related to burnout, particularly in individuals who have inadequate coping mechanisms. In your role as a new nurse, and with the competing demands for attention and the associated emotions on the job, your reservoir of coping strategies will probably run dry after a busy day. Physical exercise is a key factor in managing your stress and building personal resilience.

The physical and emotional benefits of exercise have been well documented for many years (Blaber, 2005; Centers for Disease Control and Prevention, 2009; U.S. Department of Health and Human Services, 2008). The biochemicals (endorphins) that produce a feeling of wellbeing, the tension reducing and cathartic effects of aerobic exercise, and the overall improvements in energy and cognitive functioning are but a few examples of the benefits. It's the most efficient and effective method of burning up the tensions of the day (and the calories).

Many publications since the 1960s have noted improved health and wellbeing for individuals who exercise regularly. In more recent years, cost-reduction benefits related to decreased employee sick time, injuries, and absenteeism have been demonstrated, and many health care organisations began offering onsite exercise and wellness facilities. But you don't have to exercise in an expensive facility. If your health care institution does not have an onsite gym or pool, there are other opportunities. Exploring the type of exercise that best suits you as a coping strategy is a first move. A 20-minute walk or jog after work is an excellent time to decelerate your thoughts while providing physical benefits. Some prefer dancing or aerobics classes for the added companionship and motivation. Whether taken alone or in a group, moderate or vigorous, regular activity and exercise is essential to take care of you, the caretaker (Table 9.1).

One sport that is hitting the nursing world (particularly in the United States, Canada, Australia, and New Zealand) for recreation and exercise is called *geocaching* (pronounced *geo-cashing*). Played with GPS devices, this treasure hunting game covers 192 countries throughout the world. The point is to locate hidden treasure containers outdoors and then share the experiences online. The treasure is usually something inexpensive and fun. From coins to stories, these treasures are a delight to those who participate in the hunt and hiding the treasures offers additional entertainment. The activity gets you outdoors and walking, the treasure hunt is fun and you can participate worldwide. Get started at http://www.geocaching.com.

Beginning your exercise immediately after the workday ends is important. Frequently after a busy day, getting caught up in the multiple things that you have to do (cooking, shopping, etc.) is easy and it is tempting to skip your exercise. This omission can soon become habitual. Think of your exercise time as "me time" that enables you to keep going. It provides you with respite from your work life and is a healthy transition into your personal life.

TABLE 9.1 Exercises for Sustained Performance Benefits

Moderate Intensity Exercises	**Vigorous Intensity Exercises**
Water aerobics	Swimming laps
Walking briskly	Tai Chi
Bicycling	Aerobic dancing
Tennis (doubles)	Jogging/running
Ballroom dancing	Walking briskly
General gardening	Heavy gardening
	Jumping rope
	Hiking uphill or with a heavy backpack

Source: Adapted from U.S. Department of Health and Human Services (2008).

Other Relaxing Activities

There is really no end to the kinds of activities that you can use to de-stress. It's just a matter of finding what works for you and making a commitment with yourself to engage in the activity on a regular basis. Develop a routine—both at work and for fun after work. Here are a few more ideas:

- Gardening
- Sewing
- Making jewellery
- Collecting things: searching for samples of shells, antiques, and so forth
- Attending plays, concerts, and movies
- Blogging and using Facebook, MySpace, and Twitter
- Flying
- Joining clubs outside work: cooking, book, sports, and so forth

THE STORY REVISITED

Now, let's go back and revisit Sarah's story from the beginning of the chapter. Sarah has developed a support system by building a relationship with her preceptor. Sarah now has an outlet to vent her frustrations and stresses at work and she is able to cope more effectively with the day-to-day pressures as a new graduate nurse:

> Having a support system is very important to me and helps me make sense of some of the challenging situations that I encounter at work. I have formed a bond with my preceptor who is a seasoned nurse of 20 years. She encourages me to look at the positive impact I have on patients' lives as well as look at learning opportunities that present during my clinical assignments. I called her and talked to her about the emergency incident with my patient who'd had the thyroidectomy. She listened as I reviewed the sequence of events that occurred with this situation. She reinforced that my assessment and quick actions were appropriate and saved the patient's life. I am glad I have a support system to help nurture me through this first year of practice. I definitely need a confident shoulder to lean on.

Sarah engages in other strategies to relieve the pressures from work. She enjoys taking walks in the park in her neighbourhood after work.

Walking gives her time to reflect on the positive aspects of her life and walk off the tension that sometimes occurs from her work situation. Another strategy that Sarah uses to reconnect to life and gain work–life balance is to invite friends over on weekends to play cards. Connecting with other individuals outside of work provides her time to focus on relationships outside of work and allows her to reconnect with the world around her.

CONCLUSION

On your job, you will likely feel a myriad of things in addition to fatigue. Many new graduates express feelings of being overloaded: not enough time to complete the things that they need to accomplish; feeling distress about patients, their conditions, and life situations; and comparing themselves to coworkers who seem to be so much more competent. All of these may add up to feelings of frustration and self-doubt. Without self-care, this combination can be a perfect recipe for burnout. To best help patients, nurses must practise self-care and find an appropriate balance between work life and personal life. We did not become nurses to be martyrs, yet it is difficult to flip the switch to turn off the nurse mode and begin focusing on oneself.

Throughout this chapter, we've discussed various methods of reentering our home world after leaving the work world. Finding an activity or means of leaving work behind and managing your life outside of work is a task for all of us who practice nursing. Finding a combination that fits your personal preferences and personality and offers the refreshment you need is important. Intentional and regular separation from the work world will keep you healthier and more satisfied with your nursing practice. Here, we've described several options for doing just that. It's up to you now to select and practice some activities to reenergise yourself and leave work behind. You will surely benefit!

LEARNING ACTIVITIES

Select one of the activities from the following list to experience meditation or a form of spirituality. Try the activity for a week or two and note the effect that this activity has on your stress levels. If you wish, share your experiences via a blog, email, or Twitter, or just discuss them with your fellow students.

1. Attend a local yoga class.
2. Sign up for a local meditation class.
3. Attend a religious service or a bible study class at your church.
4. Find a quiet place, play some soft music, dim the lights, and relax for 30 minutes.
5. Organise a small group of friends or fellow students to try these activities for humour and laughter.
    a. Rent and watch the movie *Patch Adams*.
    b. Go to a comedy club with a group of friends.
    c. Go to the store or library and buy or borrow a book from the humour section.
    d. Take a child to an amusement park.
6. Take three other ideas from this chapter and implement them within the next week or month and make a commitment to self-care. The priority is to care for yourself because then you will be the most beneficial nurse for your patients.

REFERENCES

Abel, M. H., & Maxwell, D. (2002). Humor and affective consequences of a stressful task. *Journal of Social and Clinical Psychology, 21*(2), 165–191.

Ablett, J. R., & Jones, R. S. P. (2007). Resilience and well-being in palliative care staff: A qualitative study of hospice nurses' experience of work. *Psycho-Oncology, 16*(8), 733–740.

Angelou, M. (1974). *Gather together in my name.* New York, NY: Random House.

Bennett, H. J. (2003). Humor in medicine: Humor and health. *Southern Medical Journal, 96*(12), 1257–1261.

Bennett, M. P., Zeller, J. M., Rosenberg, L., & McCann, J. (2003). The effect of mirthful laughter on stress and natural killer cell activity. *Alternative Therapies in Health and Medicine, 9*(2), 38–44.

Berk, L. S., Felten, D. L., Tan, S. A., Bittman, B. B., & Westengard, J. (2001). Modulation of neuroimmune parameters during the stress of humor-associated mirthful laughter. *Alternative Therapies in Health and Medicine, 7*(2), 62–76.

Blaber, A. Y. (2005). Exercise: Who needs it? *British Journal of Nursing, 14*(18), 973–975.

Casey, K., Fink, R., Krugman, M., & Propst, J. (2004). The graduate nurse experience. *Journal of Nursing Administration, 34*(6), 303–311.

Centers for Disease Control and Prevention. (2009). *Physical activity for everyone.* Retrieved from http://www.cdc.gov/physicalactivity/everyone/guidelines/index.html

Cooke, M., Holzhauser, K., Jones, M., Davis, C., & Finucane, J. (2007). The effect of aromatherapy massage with music on the stress and anxiety levels of emergency nurses: Comparison between summer and winter. *Journal of Clinical Nursing, 16*(9), 1695–1703.

De Chesnay, M. (2005). Teaching nurses about vulnerable populations. In M. de Chesnay (Ed.), *Caring for the vulnerable: Perspectives in nursing theory, practice and research* (pp. 349–356). Sudbury, MA: Jones and Bartlett, Inc.

Freud, S. (1960). *Jokes and their relation to the unconscious* (J. Strachey, Trans.). New York, NY: W. W. Norton. (Original work published 1905)

Garrity, T., Stallones, L., Marx, M. B., & Johnson, T. (1989). Pet ownership and attachment as supportive factors in the health of the elderly. *Anthrozoos, 3*(1), 35–44.

Good, M., Stanton-Hicks, M., Grass, J. A., Anderson, G. C., Lai, H. L., Roykulcharoen, V., & Adler, P. A. (2001). Relaxation and music to reduce postsurgical pain. *Journal of Advanced Nursing, 33*(2), 208–215.

Iwasaki, Y., MacKay, K., & Mactavish, J. (2005). Gender-based analyses of coping with stress among professional managers: Leisure coping and non-leisure coping. *Journal of Leisure Research, 37*(1), 1–28.

Kidd, A. H., & Kidd, R. M. (1985). Children's attitudes toward their pets. *Psychology Reports, 57*(11), 15–31.

Lazarus, R. S., & Folkman, S. (1984). *Stress, appraisal, and coping.* New York, NY: Springer.

Mahony, D. L., Burroughs, W. J., & Hieatt, A. C. (2001). The effects of laughter on discomfort thresholds: Does expectation become reality? *The Journal of General Psychology, 128*(2), 217–227.

McNicholas, J., & Collis, G. M. (2006). Animals as social supports: Insights for understanding animal assisted therapy. In A. Fine (Ed.), *Handbook on animal-assisted therapy: Theoretical foundations and guidelines for practice* (pp. 49–71). Amsterdam, The Netherlands: Elsevier.

Miller, M. A. (1995). Culture, spirituality, and women's health. *Journal of Obstetric, Gynecologic, and Neonatal Nursing, 24*(3), 257–263.

Nilsson, U., Rawal, N., & Unosson, M. (2003). A comparison of intraoperative or postoperative exposure to music—a controlled trial of the effects on postoperative pain. *Anesthesia, 58*(7), 699–703.

Svebak, S., Kristoffersen, B., & Aasarod, K. (2006). Sense of humor and survival among a county cohort of patients with end-stage renal failure: A two-year prospective study. *International Journal of Psychiatry in Medicine, 36*(3), 269-281.

Tugade, M., & Fredrickson, B. (2004). Resilient individuals use emotions to bounce back from negative emotional experiences. *Journal of Personality and Social Psychology, 86*(2), 320-333.

Tusaie, K., & Dyer, J. (2004). Resilience: A historical review of the construct. *Holistic Nursing Practice, 18*(1), 3-10.

U.S. Department of Health and Human Services. (2008). *The 2008 physical activity guidelines for Americans.* Retrieved from http://www.health.gov/paguidelines/guidelines/default.aspx#toc

U.S. Department of Health and Human Services, National Institutes of Health, & National Center for Complementary and Alternative Medicine. (2009) *Meditation* (Publication D308). Retrieved from http://nccam.nih.gov/health/meditation/meditation.pdf

Welch, V. (2009). Investing in the future: The value of volunteerism. *Urologic Nursing, 29*(4), 212-213.

Wells, D. L. (2007). Domestic dogs and human health: An overview. *British Journal of Health Psychology, 12*(1), 145-156.

Wells, D. L. (2009). Associations between pet ownership and self-reported health status in people suffering from chronic fatigue syndrome. *The Journal of Alternative and Complementary Medicine, 15*(4), 407-413.

(10) Things Just Got Really Serious: Coping in Crisis

Jane Shakespeare-Finch

INTRODUCTION

You have chosen to enter a profession that can afford you a wonderfully rich career. Within nursing are many specialty roles and many opportunities and challenges in communicating with a vast array of people, including patients and their families, peers, and management. Inherent in the role are all sorts of potential stressors, such as not having the equipment you need at a time you think you crucially need it, working with people you find difficult, shift work, lack of staffing, overcrowding—the list is sometimes seemingly endless. However, there are also obvious advantages to your role, such as meeting various people, helping ill people to recover and to feel comfortable in your care, and supporting families, patients, and colleagues. This brings me to the two primary points of this chapter.

The first point of this chapter is to understand that sometimes the challenges you may face in the health arena overwhelm your initial understanding of your capacity to cope. That is to say, there will likely be times when you feel overwhelmed or even distraught in the face of a particular situation. The second point is that these same overwhelming experiences can provide a catalyst for you to grow as a human being; to develop beyond the person you perceived yourself to be beforehand. According to Aaron Antonovsky (1985), stress is inherent in the human condition, but further to that, in your role, there is a very high possibility of traumatic experiences as well.

Acknowledge that there may come a time when you encounter a problem that is overwhelming. There are two points to note:

1. You may simply need to accept the situation.
2. From adversity can come growth.

WHAT IS TRAUMA?

The definition of a traumatic experience has two components: the nature of the event, and your response to it. In terms of the nature of the event, a traumatic event involves death or the threat of death or serious injury. In terms of your response to the event, the response is one of fear, horror, or helplessness (American Psychiatric Association, 2000). You may be the primary victim or the survivor of a trauma, or you may also be a witness to the traumatic experience of another person. For example, in your chosen career, you are privy to the intimate details of people's lives and, as a result, you share moments of great joy and, sometimes, moments of great pain. If you find yourself being overwhelmed by this experience of being witness to, or confronted by, somebody else's trauma, and you respond with fear or horror or a sense that you are helpless, your experience is called *vicarious trauma*. Vicarious trauma has the power to provide a catalyst for both distress and growth.

Several studies have examined the potential for work-related trauma to be a catalyst for nurses to develop pathology such as posttraumatic stress disorder (PTSD; e.g., Mealer, Shelton, Berg, Rothbaum, & Moss, 2007). However, other studies have examined how, in similar circumstances, health care professionals develop resilience (Ablett & Jones, 2007) and undergo posttraumatic growth (PTG; Calhoun & Tedeschi, 2006; Shakespeare-Finch, Smith, Gow, Embelton, & Baird, 2003). Many strategies can be used to deal with the difficulties mentioned in other chapters in this book. In this chapter, the focus is on cognitions—looking at how and what people think after highly aversive or traumatic experiences and finding ways in which to alter unhelpful cognitions and promote adaptive thoughts. The following vignette portrays a nurse's first experience in dealing with a crisis. That is to say, in the first instance, and for a while following, she felt completely overwhelmed by the event and doubted her capacity to cope. The chapter goes on to discuss the cognitive processes she recalls going through on her journey to weaving the experience into the story of her life.

MILLIE'S STORY

Millie was a first year nursing graduate when Mr. Ilion was brought into emergency. She had been in the emergency department for 2 months and was really enjoying the energy of the job and the variety of cases, as well as feeling a bit apprehensive about the demands she was quickly learning to face. On balance, Millie was sure this was the job for her.

Mr. Ilion looked familiar to Millie as she set about taking his vitals and asking what had happened. He said that he had experienced difficulty breathing and that his wife had called the ambulance, but that he had always looked after himself and so he was not really worried. Millie assured Mr. Ilion, his wife, and his daughter that he was going to be fine because he was now in good hands.

When Millie came back on shift the next day, she discovered that shortly after leaving the previous night, Mr. Ilion had died. Millie was shocked by the news, but was also shocked by her reaction to it. She was absolutely devastated by his death; she was not even able to suppress her emotions in front of her colleagues. Why? What was it that created a reaction of absolute gut-wrenching, vomit-inducing despair? After all, he was a patient, and patients sometimes don't make it. What Millie didn't know at the time she was telling Mr. Ilion and his family that he would be fine was that he had experienced some chest pain several times in the past and was becoming increasingly easily fatigued. Mr. Ilion had undiagnosed pulmonary hypertension. He was a positive man, enjoyed running, probably worked a bit too hard, and he had not really paid attention to the few warning signs.

Nevertheless, Millie had told them he would be fine; she looked into his daughter's eyes and said, "He will be fine."

THE SUBJECTIVE NATURE OF TRAUMA

Trauma is in the eye of the beholder. Although there are many events that are likely to be extremely traumatic to almost anyone, the thing that "rocks the boat" of one person does not necessarily create more than a ripple for another. That is why another person cannot presume to know what a *critical incident* is for someone else. Hence, it is inappropriate to think that there is only one way of coming to the aid of someone in need of support, or one way to assist yourself when your perception of the world and your place in it shifts dramatically. If the first reaction you have to an event is that it threatens your life or someone else's life, or has a threat of serious injury, and that the experience overwhelms your perception about your capacity to cope, then that event can be considered traumatic for you (American Psychiatric Association, 2000). In other words, the ways in which you have coped with the stressors of life up to that point are doubted in the immediate aftermath of trauma—in the aftermath of your response to the event. Naturally, there are also times (most often for health care professionals) when death or the threat of death does not coincide with feelings of being overwhelmed. In these situations, you are confident that you can effectively deal with the situation, including your response to it.

> Trauma is subjective. It can result from direct experience of a major critical incident. Or it can result from indirectly witnessing it.

In the story, Millie was completely overwhelmed. She could not make sense of how she felt. She just knew she was completely shattered. However, Millie was a newly qualified nurse. She had to come to terms with her experience, to learn to accept her emotions and for her to gain some sense of understanding about her intense distress at her patient's passing. Of course, the reactions Millie had are exactly that: reactions. The way we experience trauma and what we find traumatising are quite deeply engrained.

Nevertheless, that does not mean we cannot modify our reaction, learn from it, and ultimately use it for our own development. Recall the first chapter in this book. Several people who experienced extremely traumatic events but somehow managed not just to survive their ordeals but also to grow significantly were discussed. The point I want to emphasise is that an experience of trauma may provide fertile ground for understanding how best to deal with challenges to come. Let's consider Millie and the cognitive processes that followed her reaction to Mr. Ilion's death.

His presentation was not particularly disturbing, and Mr. Ilion and Millie had an immediate connection of sorts. You may well have had the experience of thinking that you have met someone before or, in some way, he or she is very familiar to you. Jung (1964) called these experiences the recognition of archetypes. He explained this phenomenon as the experience you have when someone reminds you of the archetype, or preconceived notion you have of a person in a particular role. There are many archetypes, including nurturer, warrior, innocent, and lover.

Of course, there are other theoretical explanations for Millie's feelings of knowing. Perhaps Mr. Ilion simply looked like someone she knew well enough to feel familiar with, someone she knew well enough to dismiss immediately as not being the person in front of her. Regardless of how the feeling is explained, the result is that Millie felt a connection with Mr. Illion. In the days after his death, Millie thought about him constantly, even though she didn't want to be preoccupied with thoughts of him. Nor could she get the face of his daughter out of her mind, and at unexpected times she would see his daughter's trusting eyes as Millie told her he would be okay. In the weeks that followed, Millie realised that she was struck with how much like her father Mr. Ilion looked. Therefore, it was not the patient presentation that disturbed her as much as it was the sense of familiarity she felt with him. In this case, Millie could not help but blur the lines between who this patient was and whom she *feared* he may have been. Further, she felt racked by guilt because she had told his wife and daughter he would be fine.

These insights offer some potential explanations for Millie's strong emotional connection with her patient. This sort of connection can make one person experience trauma over a particular death, whereas other health professionals have no such reaction.

> Sometimes when we make a connection with a patient, we can also feel more distressed or traumatised when things go wrong.

A large body of research attests to the experiences health care professionals find traumatic, often the times when the patient is seen in the context of their own lives and a personal connection is made (Robinson,

2002; Shakespeare-Finch & Scully, 2008). In this case, Millie felt that she knew Mr. Ilion, and she identified with his daughter. Of course, these were not conscious thoughts at the time; just a comfortable, familiar feeling.

Other situations reported by health care professionals that many find particularly disturbing include attending to a child who has been abused by a parent, a suicide or attempted suicide, and like Millie, having a sense of recognition (Robinson, 2002). For example, an intensive care paramedic once told me that a fatal case, in which he thought he recognised the hands of the patient as those of his daughter, haunted him for years. Despite being a highly qualified health care professional who readily faced horrific scenes, it took a long time for him to come to terms with the intense emotion and disruption to his thoughts that the case produced in him. Such examples remind us that even though many years in the health care arena can afford you ample opportunities to learn how to effectively deal with challenging events, you are not necessarily immune to being caught off guard and overwhelmed on occasion.

> Understand that there may be times when you will be particularly vulnerable to feeling the pain of loss or of other people's loss. Be kind to yourself. You are human and, to do your job well, you need to feel for patients and express your own feelings.

OUTCOMES AFTER TRAUMA

Trauma research has traditionally focused on the capacity of such experiences to lead to pathology like depression, anxiety, and PTSD (Hapke, Schumann, Rumpf, John, & Meyer, 2006). However, the lifetime commonality of trauma is estimated at between 49.5% and 89.6% in the general community (Breslau et al., 1998; Creamer, Burgess, & McFarlane, 2001; Kessler, Sonnega, Bromet, Hughes, & Nelson, 1995), yet there are low levels of corresponding pathology in the general community and the reality is that most people do not go on to suffer these disorders. In other words, most people are resilient to such experiences and, for some people, these experiences provide a catalyst for growth.

Chapter 1 reminded us that rising above adversity is possible. Research-based evidence bears this out. Over the past 15 to 20 years, there has been a rapid development in research that focuses on the potential for trauma to provide a springboard for growth. *Growth* refers to moving beyond the level of functioning of a person before an event. The most comprehensive model of this type of change is the model of PTG, which was proposed in the mid-1990s (Tedeschi & Calhoun, 1995, 1996) and was last refined in 2006 (Calhoun & Tedeschi, 2006).

Calhoun and Tedeschi's (2006) model of PTG posits that the types of experiences such as what Millie experienced shatter previously held assumptions about the world and a person's perceptions of himself or herself in the world. That is, we all have schemas or pictures in our minds about all sorts of things. These schemas are completely disrupted and, hence, questioned when an event creates what has been termed a "psychological earthquake" (Tedeschi, Park, & Calhoun, 1998). This psychological earthquake disrupts a person's core beliefs (Cann et al., 2010) and prompts rumination (i.e., prolonged thoughts). At first, the rumination is intrusive; you think about it when you don't want to, unwanted images come to mind, and perhaps dreams are disrupted. For some people, the nature of their dreams (nightmares) changes, but of course, this is not an inevitable part of adjusting to trauma. After a while, for most people, these symptoms of distress reduce and, in the PTG model, are replaced with effortful or purposeful ruminations. So, you may start to think about the event in a different way, try to make sense of it, bestow it with meaning, and actively engage in a process of learning through the experience (Calhoun & Tedeschi, 2006; Cann et al., 2010; Frankl, 1984; Nietzsche, 2005).

In due course, thinking about the event stops being something that you cannot control and starts to be more deliberate and purposeful. The thing is, once you have experienced a traumatic event, you cannot "unexperience" it. Imagine that your life is a tapestry, an intricate creation of colour, texture, and movement. PTG is about weaving that experience of trauma into the tapestry of your life and moving forward with new knowledge and insight as a result.

> Posttraumatic growth involves integrating the experience of trauma into your life and moving forward with new knowledge and wisdom as a result.

The tapestry of your life develops a new depth, more detail, more colour; parts may be dark, but there are also areas of light. Sounds easy, doesn't it? However, it is not. The very fact that the event was traumatic for the person means that it is anything but easy. Before I go on to talk about some processes that may lead to growth, I will take a moment to further explain what PTG is.

There are three necessary precursors, or caveats, to make explicit before such a discussion. The first is to note that growth is not an automatic by-product of trauma and does not occur for all people by any means. The second is that growth does not preclude distress. Indeed, ongoing distress is part of the PTG model. In simple terms, some days, posttrauma are good days and some days may not be. The third is that there are cultural differences in terms of what comprises growth (Weiss & Berger, 2010). However, there is also much evidence to suggest that the fundamental notion of growth is universal. For example, growth from suffering has been spoken about for millennia not only through legends and myths but also through philosophical doctrines such as Buddhism. From a Buddhist framework, it is impossible to move to a higher level of enlightenment without suffering and without assisting those who are suffering (Ho, 2005). Christian doctrines speak of God sending events to test people, the ultimate intention of which is further development. Philosophers have spoken about growth and the ways it may be achieved. For example, Friedrich Nietzsche (2005) said, and I paraphrase, that suffering ceases to be suffering when you make meaning of a situation. Likewise, Viktor Frankl (1984) spoke of meaning making as a way forward after horrendous experiences such as his time in three concentration camps during the Second World War. His faith in meaning as a vehicle for healing was realised in his development of *logotherapy* (meaning therapy).

> Numerous role models throughout history demonstrate that not only is it possible to grow after adversity, but learning from the experience can make you a better person.

Differences in cultural views of growth appear to centre around the *inter*personal as opposed to the *intra*personal notions of growth, religiosity versus spirituality, strength as a *reason for* survival rather than a *product of* survival, and so on (Ho, Chan, & Ho, 2004; Nader, Dubrow, & Stamm, 1999; Peltzer, 2000; Shakespeare-Finch & Morris, 2010). In our discussion here, we will adopt the five-factor model of growth originally developed by Tedeschi and Calhoun (1996) in the United States. The factor structure of this model has been replicated in other Western nations such as Australia (Morris, Shakespeare-Finch, Rieck, & Newbery, 2005). The five dimensions of growth are as follows (Morris et al., 2005; Tedeschi & Calhoun, 1996):

1. Developing a greater sense of personal strength
2. A new appreciation for life
3. Changes in relationships
4. A change in priorities
5. Spiritual and religious changes

The sorts of statements that trauma survivors endorse include, "I discovered that I was stronger than I thought I was," and "I have changed my priorities in life." The fact that an event is traumatic, that effort is involved in finding a resolution for your own wellbeing, that wisdom may follow, and that growth does not preclude ongoing distress are all very important points to remember. For the interested reader, please see Calhoun and Tedeschi's (2006) *Handbook of Posttraumatic Growth.* Another point to remember is that growth is not the same as resilience. Resilience refers to the idea of bouncing back following adversity and does not include the processes of adjusting to life posttrauma and developing beyond pre-event levels of functioning, which we have been discussing.

Growing After Trauma

So, how do you develop a sense of growth after trauma, and what does it mean for you when facing further difficulties in your work role and also in your personal life? Well, there are several things that can assist the posttrauma journey, and of course, there are things that can be detrimental. For example, having a social support network can be both a blessing and a curse. Having at least one person that you can confide in and that you can rely on to be there for you in times of struggle is vital (Werner & Smith, 1992). However, that person needs to be someone not only to whom you feel safe disclosing your feelings but also who validates your feelings.

For example, if Millie had admitted to a colleague that she was feeling devastated by Mr. Illion's death, the colleague may respond to her in a positive way, such as by empathising with her feelings. This validation would be a positive step towards Millie's acceptance of her feelings and could assist her to move forward. However, if Millie disclosed her feelings, the person she shared with may have said something to the effect. "But he had pulmonary hypertension and you hadn't even known him for 5 minutes." That kind of response could put Millie back quite some way on her road to acceptance of the experience and of her response to it and, hence, hinder her moving forward.

When we are traumatised, we are vulnerable and susceptible to influence. Imagine if the person making the latter statement was Millie's supervisor. Millie might then be thinking something like "What's wrong with me?" The answer is nothing is wrong with Millie other than she is in pain, because she connected with another human being who is not here anymore. Further to that, she told his wife and daughter that he would be okay. So Millie feels guilty, confused, and distressed, and that hurts. Feeling a sense of betrayal by a support network you thought would be there in times of need is an obstacle to growth and to working towards a resolution of your distressing thoughts and emotions (Shakespeare-Finch & Copping, 2006).

Therefore, expressing your emotions and having them validated by another is an important resource for growth. Expressing your thoughts and feelings rather than suppressing them is a part of the healing process. Another strategy for growth and simply for recovery from an event (i.e., resilience) is to remind yourself that, in many of life's circumstances, you cannot control what happens, but you can control your response to it. That is not to confuse the way you react (instantaneously and beyond consciousness in the first instance as discussed in Chapter 5) with the choices you make about what happens next. Some people may choose to remain angry, some will be consumed by guilt, shame, or another negative emotion, and others will decide to take the experience as an opportunity to learn. Learning more about yourself, learning new ways to view the world, your relationships, and your own capacity to deal with adversity, and other such developmental and adaptive perspectives are growth.

> Key strategies to empower your practice and achieve posttraumatic growth are to express your emotions, seek out support, talk to yourself positively about acceptance of events outside of your control, and find something that can be learned from the situation.

Your own thoughts are also largely influenced by your experiences, the people in your life, and the education you have about such matters. Hence, this chapter is designed to educate you about posttraumatic growth. We enter health professions generally because we want to be of fundamental help to other human beings and, often, be there for them in their times of greatest need and crisis. This elevated exposure to potentially traumatising events is usually treated as a potential for psychological harm. Sayings like, "If you can't handle the heat, get out of the kitchen," were common in years gone by. Thank goodness, we have come a long way since then—mostly! We now recognise not only the treatment options for those who are struggling with their mental health but also the potential for those same events that trigger considerable challenge to our coping capacity to present significant opportunities to grow and develop as human beings. Some schools of thought propose that other people's pain and our own pain are actually necessary for growth (Ho, 2005). Using a physical metaphor, if you do not stretch (use) a muscle, it will not grow; it will not develop into a bigger, stronger muscle than before. Our minds are no different, and in the profession you have chosen you are likely to be provided more opportunities to grow than those who do not occupy such roles.

A last useful cognitive strategy in dealing with trauma is to remind ourselves that it is a privilege to be there to assist others in their most vulnerable moments. Both the good days *and* the bad days make life interesting and worthwhile.

LEARNING ACTIVITIES

1. To be psychologically available to others in times of need, it is a good idea to understand something of yourself and the ways in which you deal with crisis. Knowing your strengths at a conscious level can help speed up the process of adjustment following challenge. Being conscious of your strengths can also assist you in helping others to find their own strength. A positive skill in developing and maintaining resilience is being self-aware. The following exercise in self-reflection is a useful place to start.

   Think of a difficult situation or event in your life—one that has required you to draw on your strength, resources, and strategies to successfully overcome the difficulties associated with it. Now imagine you are describing the event to someone else.

What would you say in telling them what happened for you? Please tell your story. After telling your story, try to identify the following:

a. What emotions or feelings did you have at this time?

b. Certain thoughts went through your mind. What thoughts do you remember having at the time? How did those thoughts develop over time?

c. Sometimes, our behaviours help and, at other times, they do not improve the situation or the way we feel about it. What behaviours did you engage in? Which behaviours worked well for you?

d. What strengths did you discover in yourself to deal with those previous events?

2. The following is an excerpt from a conversation I had with a survivor of the Black Saturday bushfires in Victoria, Australia, in 2009. The discussion was on the following Monday; less than 24 hours after she heard of various people in her life having been killed. In these early hours, amongst the obvious devastation, can you identify any indications of resilience and growth in the text? With the exception of me, names have been changed to protect the privacy of the people involved. This is all said in very rapid speech, which is typical when a person is in shock. Others may become silent.

I can't believe it Jane, Sue is dead and her two youngest are dead. Georgia [daughter of the person talking] has lost her best friend and I don't know where half the people are. The school has been destroyed and we've lost our animals and I have to put down the alpacas; I can't believe it. Some people are saying they'll never come back but I think we need to get together and march back into town. I'm just trying to keep the kids occupied to take their mind off it. Oh God, what are we going to do? Steve [speaker's husband] has gone back up the mountain but I can't get hold of him so I don't know what's happening. Oh God Jane, what are we going to do? They won't let us back up, but Steve managed to get through. If it wasn't for the media, we wouldn't know anything. I keep watching it to see who is alive but I can't watch it when the kids are around. I'm going to take the kids to the driving range . . .

This horrendous event killed 173 people, but that number was not known for many weeks. A year later, people are still struggling to recover, but there have also been some remarkable stories of hope and survival. An example of strength and resilience from the preceding conversation is " . . . march back into town . . . " The survivor is talking about taking control back from the fire as well as using social support to strengthen everyone's resolve. She is talking about a community spirit and of giving as well as receiving social support. In addition, the attempt to protect the children clearly indicates a presence of mind and clarity about what she feels is best for her kids. Her distraction technique of providing activities, in addition to not filling her own need for knowledge by watching the TV when the kids were about, helped to buffer them from the early stages of extreme visible distress and widespread destruction.

REFERENCES

Ablett, J. R., & Jones, R. S. P. (2007). Resilience and well-being in palliative care staff: A qualitative study of hospice nurses' experience of work. *Psycho-Oncology, 16*(8), 733–740.

American Psychiatric Association. (2000). *Diagnostic and statistical manual of mental disorders* (4th ed., text rev.). Washington, DC: Author.

Antonovsky, A. (1985). *Health, stress, and coping.* London, England: Jossey-Bass.

Breslau, N., Kessler, R. C., Childcoat, H. D., Schultz, L. R., Davis, G. C., & Andreski, P. (1998). Trauma and posttraumatic stress disorder in the community: The 1996 Detroit area survey of trauma. *Archives of General Psychiatry, 55*(7), 626–632.

Calhoun, L. G., & Tedeschi, R. G. (2006). The foundations of posttraumatic growth: An expanded framework. In L. G. Calhoun & R. G. Tedeschi (Eds.), *Handbook of posttraumatic growth: Research and practice* (pp. 3–23). Mahwah, NJ: Lawrence Erlbaum Associates.

Cann, A., Calhoun., L. G., Tedeschi, R. G., Kilmer, R. P., Gil-Rivas, V., Vishnevsky, T., & Danhauer, S. C. (2010). The Core Beliefs Inventory: A brief measure of disruption in the assumptive world. *Anxiety, Stress, and Coping, 23*(1), 19–34.

Creamer, M., Burgess, P., & McFarlane, A. C. (2001). Posttraumatic stress disorder: Findings from the Australian National Survey of Mental Health and Wellbeing. *Psychological Medicine, 31*(7), 1237–1247.

Frankl, V. (1984). *Man's search for meaning.* New York, NY: Simon and Schuster Inc.

Hapke, U., Schumann, A., Rumpf, H. J., John, U., & Meyer, C. (2006). Posttraumatic stress disorder: The role of trauma, pre-existing psychiatric disorders, and gender. *European Archives of Psychiatry and Clinical Neuroscience, 256*(5), 299–306.

Ho, S. M. Y. (2005). *Posttraumatic growth in China.* Paper presented to the American Psychological Association's 117th annual general meeting, Washington, DC.

Ho, S. M. Y., Chan, C. L. W., & Ho, R. T. H. (2004). Posttraumatic growth in Chinese cancer survivors. *Psycho-Oncology, 13*(6), 377–389.

Jung, C. G. (Ed.). (1964). *Man and his symbols.* London, England: Random House.

Kessler, R. C., Sonnega, A., Bromet, E., Hughes, M., & Nelson, C. B. (1995). Posttraumatic stress disorder in the National Comorbidity Survey. *Archives of General Psychiatry, 52*(12), 1048–1060.

Mealer, M. A., Shelton, A., Berg, B., Rothbaum, B., & Moss, M. (2007). Increased prevalence of posttraumatic stress disorder symptoms in critical care nurses. *American Journal of Respiratory and Critical Care Medicine, 175*(7), 693–697.

Morris, B. A., Shakespeare-Finch, J. E., Rieck, M., & Newbery, J. (2005). Multidimensional nature of posttraumatic growth in an Australian population. *Journal of Traumatic Stress Studies, 18*(5), 575–585.

Nader, K., Dubrow, N., & Stamm, B. H. (Eds.). (1999). *Honoring differences: Cultural issues in the treatment of trauma and loss.* Philadelphia, PA: Brunner/Mazel.

Nietzsche, F. (2005). *Thus spoke Zarathustra: A new translation by Graham Parkes.* New York, NY: Oxford Press.

Peltzer, K. (2000). Trauma symptom correlates of criminal victimization in an urban community sample, South Africa. *Journal of Psychology in Africa, South of the Sahara, the Caribbean and Afro-Latin America, 10*(1), 49–62.

Robinson, R., (2002). *Follow-up study of health and stress in ambulance services in Victoria.* Melbourne, Australia: Victorian Ambulance Crisis Counselling Unit.

Shakespeare-Finch, J. E., & Copping, A. (2006). A grounded theory approach to understanding cultural differences in posttraumatic growth. *Journal of Loss and Trauma, 11*(5), 355–371.

Shakespeare-Finch, J. E., & Morris, B. A. (2010). Posttraumatic growth in Australian populations. In T. Weiss & R. Berger (Eds.), *Transformation in context: Posttraumatic growth across cultures* (pp. 157–186). New York, NY: Wiley.

Shakespeare-Finch, J. E., & Scully, P. J. (2008). Ways in which paramedics cope with, and respond to, natural large-scale disasters. In K. M. Gow & D. Paton (Eds.), *The phoenix of natural disasters: Community resilience* (pp. 89–100). New York, NY: Nova.

Shakespeare-Finch, J. E., Smith, S. G., Gow, K. M., Embelton, G., & Baird, L. (2003). The prevalence of posttraumatic growth in emergency ambulance personnel. *Traumatology, 9*(1), 58–70.

Tedeschi, R. G., & Calhoun, L. G. (1995). *Trauma & transformation: Growing in the aftermath of suffering.* Thousand Oaks, CA: Sage Publications.

Tedeschi, R. G., & Calhoun, L. G. (1996). The Posttraumatic Growth Inventory: Measuring the positive legacy of trauma. *Journal of Traumatic Stress, 9*(3), 455–471.

Tedeschi, R. G., Park, C. L., & Calhoun, L. G. (Eds.). (1998). *Posttraumatic growth: Positive changes in the aftermath of crisis.* Mahwah, NJ: Lawrence Erlbaum Associates.

Weiss, T., & Berger, R. (Eds). (2010). *Transformation in context: Posttraumatic growth across cultures.* New York, NY: Wiley.

Werner, E., & Smith, R. (1992). *Overcoming the odds: High-risk children from birth to adulthood.* New York, NY: Cornell University Press.

(11) Now It's My Turn: Becoming the Image of the Good Leader

Linda Shields

INTRODUCTION

Much has been written on theories of leadership and what makes a good leader. In this chapter, I am going to tell you of some who have been (and still are) great leaders in nursing, and I will weave into their stories various aspects of leadership theory that have resonance for me. As such, this chapter will have something of a personal timbre, but I will try to keep it light. In that spirit, I will make a start.

Lord Byron said that "when we think we lead we most are led" (Byron, 1821). Although Byron was never known for his humility, such sentiments do indicate one of the essences of a good leader. Leadership theories have been around forever. The Bible is full of them, and quotes about leadership by ancient writers such as Lao-Tzu (Shun, 1995) and Homer (Taplin, 1986) are still commonly used. It is not my intention to bore you with a string of clichés about either leadership or leaders. If one cannot name a dozen well-known leaders, then surely, one needs to read more, and in these times of instant gratification of curiosity through Google or Bing, there is no excuse for not being able to name at least a few. Have I become a leader? I hope so, though others will be better able to judge that than I. I will discuss some of the characteristics of a good leader as I see them. I will tell you of some wonderful leaders I have known, and what makes them leaders. Most of these people will not make the "most famous people" list, but they are leaders, nonetheless. In describing them, I hope we will all learn how we can model their characteristics to help us become leaders as well. I call them my "nursing heroes."

PROFESSOR ROGER WATSON

The International Council of Nurses (ICN) is, of course, our leading international body. For many years, it was led by Dr. Margretta Styles (Basu, 2005), who, when she was still the president, I heard say, "Nursing will know it has succeeded when a nurse is awarded a Nobel Prize." Because the Nobel Prize is the penultimate accolade for intellectual achievement, it is good for nurses to strive towards such a laudable goal. Roger Watson (Figure 11.1) is a modern leader who, as Editor-in-Chief of the *Journal of Clinical Nursing*, has developed the journal to its status as one of the top five international journals in nursing. He recently said that a nurse may never be able to win a Nobel Prize because nursing is such a hybrid of philosophies; there is no one agreed definition of nursing, and it

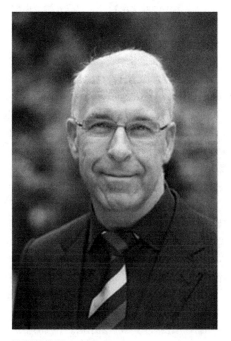

FIGURE 11.1   Professor Roger Watson.

is neither a uniquely scientific nor artistic endeavour (Watson, 2008). Nursing is made up of such a range of activities, theories, and constructs that it is hard to combine into a single entity. Hence, the Nobel Prize, which is awarded in specific disciplines such as medicine, science, or literature, may not fit with nursing. Watson does, however, conclude that this "glitch" should never preclude us from striving to win the Nobel Prize and that personal enterprise and striving for the highest standards and goals should be an integral part of nurses' ethics and motivation.

(An important leadership strategy is to assert your own
beliefs even if others may criticize you.)

Many people disagreed with Watson's remarks, and for some time, he received correspondence from other nurses that was, shall we say, not constructive. Nevertheless, he showed great leadership in saying what he did, in making us sit up, take notice, and reflect on what nursing is all about and our part in it. A willingness to put oneself in line for criticism and, more negatively, personal attack (there are many people who cannot discern the difference between the two) is a characteristic of a leader that I personally applaud and try to emulate. Roger Watson's web page can be found at: http://www.sheffield.ac.uk/snm/staff/rwatson/profile.html.

Paul Keating, a former Prime Minister of Australia (Keating & National Press Club [Australia], 1990), once said, "Leadership is not about being nice. It's about being right and being strong." Some leaders are less public but have wonderful characteristics that can endear and infuriate at the same time. Although many of us strive to be seen as "nice" people, occasionally, there are some who lead by bringing to our attention issues that, although they need to be addressed, may cause intense irritation. Such a leader was Sister Mary Dorothea.

SISTER MARY DOROTHEA SHEEHAN, R. S. M.

The first time I met Sister Mary Dorothea, I saw an energetic woman in her early 60s who spoke in a strong and determined voice about what she expected of me as a new employee of her hospital. As a Sister of Mercy (Institute of the Sisters of Mercy, Australia, 2007), Sister Mary Dorothea had devoted her life to the care of children at the Mater Hospital, a large

Catholic hospital in Brisbane, Australia (Shields, 1999). When I went to work there, Dot, as she was affectionately known, had been director of nursing (under the position's several titles) for many years. She had begun life in a small country town, completed her nursing training (as it was called in those days) at the Mater Hospital, and then joined the convent in 1938. She ruled with a fist of iron in a velvet glove; her determination to make her hospital a family-friendly place for her small patients was matched only by her commitment to making it a safe, secure, and good place to work for her nurses. Dot knew all our names (even those, who like me, worked permanent night duty). She may not have known our children's names, but there was nothing she liked better than to take us aside and find out how they were getting on at school and, most importantly, she listened and remembered what we told her. Then at the next encounter, she asked salient questions about our families.

Working in a children's hospital is a very rewarding job, but can have its down side. The death of a child is always distressing and, on night duty, seemed to be even more so. One of my fondest memories of Dot (and the other nuns who worked with her) is indicative of the care she gave to her nursing staff. When we had a child dying on the ward, we would, of course, support the parents to the best of our abilities. Dot and the two Sisters of Mercy who were her nursing supervisors (the term used at the time), Sister Marie and Sister Collette, would leave their beds, come into the ward, and make cups of tea and coffee for the nursing staff.

> Another leadership strategy is to demonstrate care through compassionate action.

As well as having a huge compassion for her charges, Dot was a fighter, but always in the nicest way possible, and this extended to her advocacy for children and their families. She was notorious amongst the hospital board members for bringing her advocacy to the fore at the end of a discussion in an executive meeting. After a long discussion of some point about running the hospital, just when everyone thought a decision had been made, Dot would say, "Ah, yes, but children are different!" and the discussion would have to start all over again.

What did I learn from Dot? Firstly, that good manners can be assertiveness in another guise. Next, that determination about something one thinks is right will help one be assertive, and that advocacy for others, as well as for oneself, is an important part of a nurse's role. However, Dot's most important lesson to me was the value of compassion, and how it is important not just for the children, families, and patients who come to us for care, but for those with whom one works. This lesson of compassion is especially important if one is a leader and (dare I say "or"?) in a management role.

While Dot was a fighter at a time when resources were (relatively) plentiful, my next "hero" was a leader in a time when all resources were being used to fight a war.

DAME MAUD McCARTHY

Emma Maud McCarthy (Figure 11.2) was born in Sydney in 1859, the first child in the large family of a prominent solicitor, and her maternal uncle was chief justice of Victoria, Sir William á Beckett (McCarthy, 1986). In

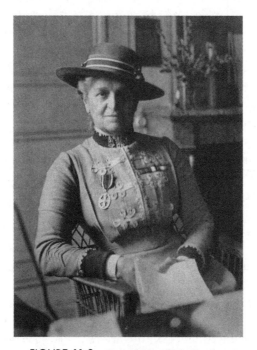

FIGURE 11.2   Dame Maud McCarthy.
Source: Published with permission of
Trustees of the Army Medical Services
Museum, Aldershot, UK.

1891, giving her age as 28 (she was older than 30), Maud, as she was known, began her training as a nurse at The London Hospital in Whitechapel. Her probationer report describes her as "a lady," "wanting courage," "needing more force of character" (The London Hospital, 1894). However, by 1894, she had been made sister and along with six other sisters from The London Hospital was chosen to go to the war in South Africa as Princess Alexandra's Military Nursing Contingent. She served there from 1899 to 1902, and was awarded the Royal Red Cross, and the Queen's and the King's Medal.

In 1902, Queen Alexandra's Imperial Military Nursing Service (QAIMNS) was formed (Piggott, 1990). With high standards of professional knowledge and experience required, these nurses were experts in modern nursing techniques. An inherent part of their work and training was a high level of compassion towards the servicemen whom they served. In 1903, Maud McCarthy joined QAIMNS as a matron and served at the Royal Victoria Military Hospital Netley, then Millbank Military Hospital. In 1910, she was appointed a principal matron in the British War office.

When the First World War began in 1914, Maud McCarthy was promoted to Matron-in-Chief for France and Flanders. She left England on the first ship for the battlefields of the Western front and was responsible for the administration of nursing facilities throughout the Somme campaign. Her authority covered nurses from Britain, Australia, Canada, New Zealand, South Africa, India, and the United States (Light, 2009).

After the armistice was signed on 11 November 1918, Maud McCarthy left France only after she had closed down her headquarters and made sure all her nurses were home safely. She remained Matron-in-Chief of QAIMNS and was decorated many times by the United Kingdom, France, Belgium, and America (McCarthy, 1986), including the award of Dame Grand Cross.

After the war, Dame Maud McCarthy was Matron-in-Chief of the Territorial Army Nursing Service from 1920 to 1925. She was made a Lady of Grace of the Grand Priory of the Hospital of St. John of Jerusalem in England in 1919 and died in 1949 in London. Sadly, now, in her own country—Australia—little is known about this great leader. She was much loved and respected by her nurses, by military confreres and commanders, and by the patients, with whom she had a surprising amount of interaction, given her lofty position. Dame Maud McCarthy was a true leader, and it remains an indictment on Australian and British nursing that she is so poorly remembered.

> Important leaders in nursing may sometimes be over-
> looked because of our culture of doing without reflect-
> ing, celebrating, and hailing our own. One key strategy
> you can take on is to promise to notice and validate
> nursing leaders you value.

Dame Maud McCarthy was a great organiser and administrator, which, of course, are valuable leadership qualities. But her concern for her nurses and the men for whom they cared showed that under the tight military discipline, there lurked the same sort of compassion that Sister Mary Dorothea was able to demonstrate openly. My next hero had to hide all her compassion, ethics, and actions because her leadership put her life in danger on a daily basis.

MARIA STROMBERGER

Maria Stromberger (Figure 11.3) was also active in wartime and, similarly to Dame Maud, she is not well remembered. Her leadership qualities were very different from the other nurses I am describing, because they had to be covert, subtle, and draw no attention. Maria Stromberger was born in 1869 and, like Dame Maud, did not commence her nursing train-ing until she was in her 30s (Benedict, 2006). While working in an infec-tious diseases hospital in Königshütte in Poland in 1942, she heard stories of terrible happenings at a place in Poland called Auschwitz. Maria Strom-berger, much to the disquiet of her sister, applied for and got the job as head nurse in the Revier, or camp hospital, for SS soldiers at Auschwitz. The Revier was in proximity to the main crematorium and gas cham-bers, so she saw and heard for herself what was occurring there. She resolved that it was her humanitarian duty to try to help as many prison-ers as she could. Until she herself became ill in 1944, Maria Stromberger smuggled in food, medicine, guns, and ammunition for the prisoners, and smuggled out letters, reports, and film of what was happening, so the world could be told of the horrors taking place. Remarkably, she was not caught—perhaps, we must assume that she was highly intelligent as well as highly moral because the consequences of being caught would have been not just death but prolonged torture. Ironically, after the war,

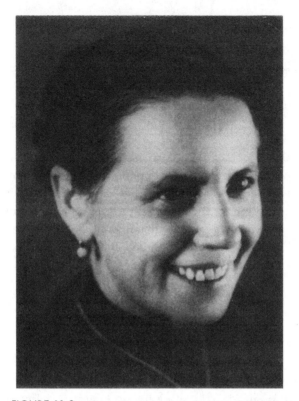

FIGURE 11.3   Maria Stromberger. *Source:* Published
with permission of Archiv der Landeshauptstadt Bregenz.

she was imprisoned by the French who thought she was a Nazi, and it
was not until Polish and Jewish prisoners and former members of the
Polish Resistance presented testimony of her courageous work that she
was freed (Benedict, 2006). Today, little is known about this woman
who risked so much.

What life was like for Maria Stromberger is difficult to imagine,
although after the war she never nursed again, choosing instead to work
in a textile factory. The enormity of what she did deserves far more
recognition than she has received, and her leadership qualities were of
the highest order, particularly those surrounding moral choice, ethical
actions, and being true to oneself and one's beliefs. Obviously, Maria
Stromberger could receive no accolades for her work at that time, but the
fact that she is so little known now is very sad. Perhaps she personifies
the humility characteristic of the greatest leaders.

While Maria Stromberger achieved much covertly, we now live in a world where leadership achievements can be won openly in a free world. My next hero has been able to achieve much by leading people to work together, for the benefit of the nursing profession as a whole and paediatric nursing in particular.

[Leadership involves courage and principled action.]

JAN PRATT

Jan Pratt is a quiet achiever, who, while nursing director of a large metropolitan community child health service, has managed to bring into being the Australian College of Children and Young People's Nurses (2009a). As with many organisations in Australia, all the Australian states and territories had separate paediatric nursing organisations, some of which had been in place for decades. Historically, the separate states of Australia have been largely autonomous, with separate governing bodies, populations amongst whom rivalry has existed (especially around that Australian "cultural entity," the sports team), and separate health systems. Paediatric nursing suffered from the state-related jingoism that was often a hamper to effective communication with consequent negative effects on nursing as a profession and, ultimately, on patients and clients within the health services. Jan Pratt sought to change all that and, in the long term, improve care for children and families.

Such an endeavour was fraught with danger. Each state thinks that its institutions do things better than the others, with traditions individual to each state and with the idea that each state is different. In 1979, Bob Hawke, who was the prime minister from 1983 to 1991, said that Australia was the most overgoverned country in the world (Hawke, 1979), and this certainly was reflected in the number of paediatric nursing organisations. Jan was determined to join them together, to bring all paediatric (child health, adolescent, young people, neonatal, acute care, etc.) nurses to the table. Only by sundering the barriers between states, and by allowing a free exchange of ideas unhampered by artificial boundaries, would the health of children be best served.

In 2008, the Australian College of Children and Young People's Nurses was promulgated, with Dr. Jan Pratt as its first president

(Australian College of Children and Young People's Nurses, 2009b). Have all the states come on board? Well, not quite, but then, Rome wasn't built in a day, and Jan Pratt's quiet determination will continue to influence the increasing professionalism of paediatric nursing in Australia. Jan Pratt's leadership attributes include a wonderful ability to break down communication barriers, to make people want to work with each other, to reflect on their own actions and abilities, and to question. One of her strongest leadership qualities is a quietly effective positive criticality, which she uses to promote people's awareness of their own actions and decisions.

> Some leaders are quiet achievers, enacting change by showing respect for others, self-belief, and never wavering in asking questions to produce reforms.

Well, now I have presented my heroes, how do they fit into the expansive and comprehensive theories that have been written about leadership?

RESEARCH ON LEADERSHIP IN NURSING

Leadership theories abound—in fact, the paper used to publish them must have contributed significantly to global warming! A Google search of "leadership characteristics" yielded more than 65,000 hits. The ICN has published a book on leadership for nurses, and they promote the following characteristics as necessary for the "nurse leader": "vision and strategic thinking, external awareness, influence, motivation, confidence, trust, political skill, review, change and renewal of self and others, teamwork, partnerships, and alliances" (Shaw, 2007, pp. 36–37). A study of nurse executive directors in the United Kingdom (Kirk, 2009) found that they thought that their leadership qualities included appropriate use of power, effective communication, knowledge of nursing, human management skills, vision, and an ability to take a total organisation view, quality management, an astuteness about business, effective multidisciplinary collaboration, the ability to support nurses under their control, a delivery focus, political awareness, and courage. A grounded theory study of conflicts that leaders faced in Swedish nursing included ethical stress when faced with conflicting aspects of their leadership abilities and expectations (Dellve & Wikström, 2009). American leaders found that to implement leadership training in an African country, leaders needed an understanding of the multicultural aspects of both nursing and leadership and a robust ability to consult and collaborate (Lacey-Haun & Whitehead, 2009). A leadership issue that faces many of us who work in research is the thorny one of increasing research capacity amongst clinical nurses. Henderson, Winch, and Holzhauser (2009) found that leadership strategies in the research arena need to be well resourced, that a solid infrastructure that can form a reference point for those potentially interested in research is required and that effective monitoring and evaluation systems are necessary.

All of these findings are sound, and I could go on at length, but readers will be able to pursue any further reading about leadership in nursing at their leisure. I will now explain what I personally see as the qualities and characteristics of a good leader, and see what my heroes can show us.

Courage

Some of the preceding theorists have mentioned this quality. Maria Stromberger obviously had it in bucketsful. But how much courage did Roger Watson have to take the *Journal of Clinical Nursing* to the next level of development? Although exciting for him, it required considerable change. Additionally, competition from a couple of other highly regarded nursing journals that were much further developed than the *Journal of Clinical Nursing* was strong. Jan Pratt had to be very courageous when she challenged the traditionalists in the state-based paediatric nursing organisations and must have had many sleepless nights. Courage may not be something that can be learned; perhaps the neuroscientists and geneticists will one day find a gene or brain structure responsible for the characteristic "courage." However, one can become *conditioned* to courage. If you do one brave act, then sometimes (not always) it becomes easier to do another, and so on. However, reading about Victoria Cross winners, those whose bravery in battle has won them the highest of accolades, many will say that they do not regard themselves as particularly courageous. Rather, they acted on the spur of the moment when they saw others in trouble (Vasak, 2010).

Willingness to Take Risks

This character goes hand in hand with courage, and again, of my exemplars, Maria Stromberger sits at the top. She risked her life every day she was in Auschwitz. A good leader must be prepared to take a risk and celebrate, or suffer, the consequences. Not every risk will work out, and you must pick yourself up, dust yourself off, and start all over again, as the song goes. Risks do not always have the magnitude of those that Maria Stromberger faced. For us, they are more often centred on the decisions we make and the actions we take. But never to take a risk means nothing is ever tried, nothing is ever invented, and nothing develops. Life would be very boring without taking risks. Had Jan Pratt not taken a risk when she contacted paediatric nursing organisations in the other states, the Australian College of Children and Young People's Nurses would not have been created. A risk going wrong can mean learning from one's mistakes. I once took a job in another country, and it turned out to be a really bad move. However, I learned a lot about that country and nursing in it. Most importantly, I learned about myself, as I found strengths I had not realised I possessed. Although it was not very nice at that time, I would not have missed it for the world!

Toughness

Some might call this resilience, or perhaps determination, and maybe it is a combination of those qualities. You have to be tough to be a leader of any kind, but it's worth it. Imagine the good feeling when you have persevered, when you know you are doing something right, and you are determined that you are going to do the right thing. Dame Maud McCarthy had to be very tough to deal with the male officers of that time—think of all those crusty British generals! The position of matron-in-chief had a lot of clout, but we can safely assume that many of those men who, although they may never have come under her direct control, had to answer to her in other ways were not always happy about doing so. One aspect of Dame Maud's command that is found repeatedly in reports and correspondence about her was her advocacy for "her nurses." She felt a personal responsibility to ensure their safety and comfort while they were active front line participants in the bloodiest conflict in history.

Determination is part of toughness, but it may not always be necessary to be tough when determination is called for. Perhaps *wily* might be more appropriate: If you can't get over a mountain, then find a way around it.

Making and Learning From Mistakes

I once heard a radio broadcast in which a man who had been appointed director of a research facility funded by Bill Gates said that Gates told him that if he wasn't making mistakes, then he wasn't doing his job. Although I cannot find this reference, I have found one of Gates' sayings: "Failure is a great teacher" (Gates, 2004). I am certain all of my heroes have made many mistakes, and their leadership is exemplified in the fact that they persisted and succeeded, having learned from their mistakes.

Tolerance and Celebration of Difference

The world is a much smaller place today than it was for Dame Maud or Maria Stromberger, or even for Sister Mary Dorothea. We are very lucky in that we can travel to other countries readily, and others can visit us. In addition, we can easily learn about other people through the mass media. This ability should have led to more tolerance, and perhaps it has; after all, tolerance was sadly lacking in the world when Maria Stromberger was nursing. As leaders, nurses are well placed to celebrate difference because people of all races and creeds come to us for care; in fact, we are some of the most fortunate human beings because of our abilities to help others. Tolerance and an awareness of the needs of others are surely characteristics of a good leader. Perhaps all nurses are leaders because these qualities are inimical to nursing.

Compassion

A good leader who is aware of the needs of others must have compassion. Sister Mary Dorothea and her confreres in the Sisters of Mercy were, almost by definition, compassionate women. Dot's ability to be touched by the children in her care and her dogged determination to ensure they received the very best care were always present. Her compassion for both the children and their families was the driving force in her life. Dot retired just at the time when HIV and AIDS was emerging, and so, driven by the compassion that was such a part of her calling, she left the children's hospital and set up a care home for young men with HIV or AIDS when others in the community were frightened of doing so.

Humility

Using clichés in writing a chapter on leadership would be all too easy and I have tried to avoid them thus far. However, to describe humility, I find that I can no longer resist, and so must present the following pairs of leaders who, roughly, were contemporaries of each other: Jesus Christ and Julius Caesar, Thomas Jefferson and Napoleon Bonaparte, Mahatma Ghandi and Winston Churchill, and Nelson Mandela and Margaret Thatcher. All have been great leaders, but it is those with humility—Jesus, Jefferson, Ghandi, and Mandela—who, in my opinion, are the greatest. All my leaders have this defining quality, but my description of Dot providing cups of tea for the nurses who were supporting the parents of a dying child perhaps best exemplifies humility in practice. Unless a leader has humility, he or she cannot lead effectively.

> Courage, willingness to take risks, toughness, making and learning from mistakes, tolerance and celebration of difference, compassion, and humility—qualities you can develop to empower your practice.

CONCLUSION

In conclusion, leadership is about other people—after all, who does one lead? Nurses are in an ideal situation to lead others, but within nursing itself, we need good leaders. To be a good leader, one needs vision, strategic thinking, motivation, confidence and determination, trust, political skill, courage and a willingness to take risks, strength, an ability to reflect on and learn from mistakes, compassion, and, most importantly, humility. The examples presented here, those whose lives were spent as leaders in the service of others—Dame Maud McCarthy, Maria Stromberger, and Sister Mary Dorothea—and those who are still nursing leaders today—Roger Watson and Jan Pratt—show special qualities that have enabled them to motivate, encourage, support, and, at times, succour other nurses.

Why is this important? Without leaders, we will not, as a profession, as humans, or as a civilisation and culture, move forward. You, the readers of this book, are either potential or existing leaders. I trust you have gleaned some information, tips, and advice on your leadership that will enable you to carry yourselves and others through this wonderful profession of nursing.

LEARNING ACTIVITIES

1. Interview someone you think is a very good leader. Record the interview and write it up as a paper for a nursing journal. Add comments on the leadership qualities you see in this person that you would wish to emulate.
2. Find classes on leadership at your local university, in schools other than nursing (for example, in a business school). Ask if you can attend on a casual basis to learn what other disciplines regard as leadership qualities.
3. Start a discussion group at your workplace. Seek executive permission if you need to, book a room, send out email messages with the topic (pick one dear to your heart), and then guide the discussion around it.

REFERENCES

Australian College of Children and Young People's Nurses. (2009a). *ACCYPN - Promoting excellence in health care for children and young people.* Retrieved from http://www.accypn.org.au/

Australian College of Children and Young People's Nurses. (2009b). *Board members.* Retrieved from http://www.accypn.org.au/members-area/governance-information/board/

Basu, J. (2005, November 29). Former UCSF Nursing Dean Margretta Styles dies at age 75. *UCSF News Office Media Advisory*. Retrieved from http://news.ucsf.edu/releases/former-ucsf-nursing-dean-margretta-styles-dies-at-age-75/

Benedict, S. (2006). Maria Stromberger: A nurse in the resistance in Auschwitz. *Nursing History Review*, *14*, 189–202.

Byron, G. G. (1821). *The Two Foscari*: Act II, Sc.1, p. 63. London, England: John Murray.

Dellve, L., & Wikström, E. K. (2009). Managing complex workplace stress in health care organizations: Leaders' perceived legitimacy conflicts. *Journal of Nursing Management*, *17*(8), 931–941.

Gates, W. (2004, January 26). *Advancing enterprise*. Keynote address presented at the Enterprising Britain Conference. Retrieved from http://www.hm-treasury.gov.uk/ent_entconf_gates.htm

Hawke, R. J. L. (1979). *The resolution of conflict* (1979 Boyer Lectures). Sydney, Australia: Australian Broadcasting Commission.

Henderson, A., Winch, S., & Holzhauser, K. (2009). Leadership: The critical success factor in the rise or fall of useful research activity. *Journal of Nursing Management*, *17*(8), 942–946.

Institute of the Sisters of Mercy, Australia. (2007). [Home page]. Retrieved from http://www.mercy.org.au/

Keating, P., & National Press Club (Australia). (1990). *Paul Keating address at the National Press Club, Canberra, May 9, 1990* [Sound recording]. National Press Club, Canberra.

Kirk, H. (2009). Factors identified by nurse executive directors as important to their success. *Journal of Nursing Management*, *17*(8), 956–964.

Lacey-Haun, L. C., & Whitehead, T. D. (2009). Leading change through an international faculty development programme. *Journal of Nursing Management*, *17*(8), 917–930.

Light, S. (2009). *War diary: Matron-in-chief, British Expeditionary Force, France and Flanders*. Retrieved from http://www.scarletfinders.co.uk/110.html

The London Hospital. (1894). Emma Maud McCarthy, September 1891–October 1894. In *London Hospital Probationer Register*. Royal London Hospital Archives, Reference LH/N/1/4.

McCarthy, P. M. (1986). McCarthy, Dame Emma Maud (1859–1949). *Australian dictionary of biography online edition*. Retrieved from http://www.adb.online.anu.edu.au/biogs/A100210b.htm

Piggott, J. (1990). Queen Alexandra's Royal Army Nursing Corps. In B. Horrocks (Ed.), *Famous regiments*. London, England: Leo Cooper, Ltd.

Shaw, S. (2007). *International Council of Nurses: Nursing leadership*. Oxford, UK: Blackwell Publishing.

Shields, L. (1999). Celebrating nursing achievement: Sister Mary Dorothea Sheehan RSM 1916–1999. *Neonatal, Paediatric and Child Health Nursing, 2*(4), 5–7.

Shun, K. (1995). Lao-Tzu. In T. Hondereich (Ed.), *The Oxford companion to philosophy.* Oxford, UK: Oxford University Press.

Taplin, O. (1986). Homer. In J. Boardman, J. Griffin, & O. Murray (Eds.), *The Oxford history of the classical world.* Oxford, UK: Oxford University Press.

Vasak, L. (2010, January 4). Just doing my job, says VC winner Mark Donaldson. *The Australian.* Retrieved from http://www.theaustralian.com.au/news/nation/just-doing-my-job-says-vc-winner-mark-donaldson/story-e6frg6nf-1225815745839

Watson, R. (2008). Editorial: Will there ever be a Nobel Prize in nursing? *Journal of Clinical Nursing, 17*(5), 565–566.

(12) Looking Forward

*Margaret McAllister
and John B. Lowe*

Now it's time to recall the imagery exercise we had you complete at the start of the book. On the first day of your new job, the first person you met was a rude and unhappy team leader—stressed because she was short of two nurses and the ward was extremely busy. Remember we gave you three choices and you had to decide. Would you leave now before any more damage to your psyche could be inflicted? Go back into the thick of it, steeled by your ability to model yourself on that callous but competent team leader? Or reflect and apply the resilience strategies you have learned about?

The dilemma of these three choices is one that many nurses have faced in their careers and, for many, several times. Too many new graduates choose the first option and leave nursing in their first year of practice. Although it is hard, data remain elusive, it is estimated that in Australia, 20% of new nurses leave the profession after being in the workforce for only 1 year (National Nursing and Nursing Education Taskforce [N3ET], 2005). In North America, that figure is 27% (American Association of Colleges of Nursing [AACN], 2009). In fact, every country across the world is experiencing a nursing shortage. The crisis is global. The good news is that the health care sector of the economy in most developed countries is growing. As a nurse, if you are competent and maintain currency in your skills, you can confidently predict that you will be guaranteed a job for life.

We doubt you would admit to choosing the second option—that you decided to soldier on, and use the coping strategies observed in the apparently stronger people around you, despite the fact that these coping mechanisms were damaging to self and others. However, this is a common

167

reality within the health workforce. Nurses are subject to significant amounts of bullying, intimidation, and violence. We doubt that any nurses begin their careers consciously intending to become bullies. Yet, this is the reality. In Australia, the Australian Safety and Compensation Council (ASCC; 2007) reported that stress costs the economy $1.3 billion annually. The most common categories compensated were, in descending order, work pressure, harassment, exposure to violence, then other mental state factors, traumatic events, and finally, suicide or attempted suicide.

> Too many nurses leave the profession early in their career—hurt by adverse events, alienated by an impersonal or uncaring workplace. You can make a difference to this culture by being positive, surrounding yourself with people who care about you, and enacting small changes that break down bullying.

Nurses have a much higher rate of compensation than any other professional or paraprofessional group in health care (Peterson, 2007) and appear to suffer the most burnout. Interestingly, however, this stress is rarely related to patient problems (Regan, Howard, & Oyebode, 2009). We can attribute some of the stress to high work demands, made higher when dissatisfied nurses leave, thus, creating more work for their remaining colleagues; the need to learn new technologies; the need to work under increasingly intensified schedules; and having to respond to emergencies. However, some of the difficulties are self-made. Because nurses comprise 50% of the health workforce, the people responsible for managing workloads, resolving conflicts, and easing tension are very likely to be nurses. As you learned in our first story, even team leaders can feel a lack of control in their job, which can trigger stress and an unconscious use of defensive strategies. Instead of venting about the stress at the source, our team leader displaced it onto a safer target—you! Stress then continued to flow on to you, the people on whom you later vented, and so on; thus, continuing the cycle we know as horizontal violence in nursing. One or 2 years down the track, after experiencing this kind of working relationship every day, you may quite possibly unconsciously mirror the same coping style. Thus, you unconsciously become the image of the gruff but efficient nurse and unintentionally intimidate or frighten students and new graduates—putting some of them off nursing for life!

As Freire (1972) explained, horizontal violence is nonphysical intra-group conflict that is manifested in overt and covert behaviours of hostility. Horizontal violence is a characteristic of oppressed groups who have a sense of powerlessness and perceived inability to resolve their tension or problems directly with the oppressor.

> Unconscious patterns of behaviour are those that create the greatest damage. A key strategy to empower your practice is to be a *mindful practitioner*—conscious of your feelings, conscious of your actions.

But of course there are other behaviours to choose from when faced with stress, harassment, or interpersonal conflict. Recall Chapter 2 and imagine what Florence Nightingale or Mary Seacole might have done when faced with a workplace bully. Very likely they would have responded assertively. They would certainly not have internalised the negative feelings and would have moved on to complete the real work of seeing to the health and wellbeing of their patients. They embodied the third option—using resilience strategies to cope with the issues and to cultivate a happier, more productive workplace culture.

We have seen other resilience strategies illustrated in short stories throughout this book. At some later time in your career, recalling and applying these strategies will be important for your wellbeing. One of the huge benefits of storytelling for learning is that it is far easier to remember a well-told story than it is to remember lists, or facts, or figures.

> Stories can embody lessons and, if they are rich, you will remember them for life. To help future nursing students and colleagues, share the stories that motivated and inspired you.

Recall Jenny and her shoes, the patient from whom Andrew Estefan seems to have learned valuable lessons, helping him (and us) to think ethical issues through clearly and rationally, and so avoid taking the staff scepticism and cynicism to heart. Without these ethical reasoning skills, nurses are vulnerable to feeling the tension of dilemmas and simply do not know how best to respond.

Maura MacPhee provided a memorable counterpoint to our first story of insensitivity by relaying a story that shows what happens when a new graduate is welcomed by a supportive colleague. She explained that growing confidence leads to competence, and such productivity can be disseminated if positive role models abound in our workplaces. However, if a colleague is impatient or is rude to you, the impact does not have to lead to a cycle of hostility and workplace negativity. As Mary Katsikitis and Rachael Sharman explained, we have different reactive styles to events, and in our work role, we can all challenge and replace unhelpful or ineffective cognitions.

Not only can we challenge and replace our own cognitive distortions, we can also positively influence others' beliefs. When we suspend our own biases and expectations, and listen closely to other people, they will feel that their concerns have been heard. Additionally, you aren't simply confirming your own preconceived judgements and expectations. These insights were discussed in Chapter 6 by Natoshia Askelson, Mary Aquilino, and Shelly Campo. Read their chapter again, whenever you find yourself attributing reasons for other peoples' disappointing or upsetting behaviour to a single source. Nurses work in very busy environments, with many colleagues, each with their own pressing job to do. When conflict or tension occurs, rather than take a blaming approach to the individual, try to reflect on possible sources of rising tension. Appreciate that most of the time in health care, good people are trying their best to complete a very hard job.

Do you remember Dr. White causing Mary to leave sobbing into her handkerchief in Chapter 7? Tony Warne and Sue McAndrew's chapter explains that nurses work in an environment that is often highly emotionally charged. The nursing role involves the intertwining of a professional and a personal self. We don't leave our own personality or our values at home when we start the working day, and nor do our teammates. One reason that workplace tension develops, Warne and McAndrew argue, is because team members come to work with differing priorities, and not all of these priorities are familiar to other team members.

Let us give you an example: A client with schizophrenia finds it hard to maintain full employment. He is referred to an occupational therapist for assessment. The team finds it puzzling when the therapist suggests she spend a morning at the beach with this client. The therapist can't understand why the team is scoffing at her. How would you understand this situation? The point is that not all clinicians take the same view of the patient's problem as a nurse might. Furthermore, team members can learn a lot from each other about how to care for a patient holistically. In

the work environment, nurses are more likely to find their role rewarding when they can appreciate their own contribution as well as their
limitations and learn to appreciate the richness of difference.

Remember, you don't have to struggle alone to find meaning in these
challenges. Debra Jackson, Glenda McDonald, and Lesley Wilkes explained
the value of workplace supports. In Chapter 8 we met Kylie, a nurse who
was feeling so lonely and isolated at work that it was overwhelming for her.
Do you recall how she managed to turn this situation around? Answer:
through joining a professional support network and asking an admired colleague to be a mentor, so that doubts and uncertainties could be shared
and, together, solutions could be found. Professional networks can provide
a safe venue for discussing interpersonal problems productively. For example, if you are experiencing unfairness, then once it is revealed within the
group, the members can name the problem, validate their feelings, and collaborate on rectifying the situation. Remember, collaborative action is
much more effective than working alone on an entrenched problem.

In addition, when the busy day is over, as Jane Brannan, Mary de
Chesnay, and Patricia Hart helpfully remind us in Chapter 9, nurses need
to relax, unwind, and get on with living the other parts of their lives to
be fulfilled, happy, connected, and valued human beings.

Never forget, though, that nursing, like all of the health professions, is
difficult work. There will be times when even your best relaxation measures
won't help you to sleep at night. There will be grief and heartache ahead
because nursing is about caring for people when they are at their most vulnerable. Nurses work at the scene of the accident. They are there through
the night when reality hits the client facing an uncertain or frightening
prognosis. They are also standing at the door when clients are discharged,
only to greet another client in need, in pain, in another health care crisis.
Many nurses thrive in this dynamic environment, but sometimes we can be
caught by surprise and be wounded by events to which we thought ourselves immune. Recall Millie's story told by Jane Shakespeare-Finch in Chapter 10. Many stories like Millie's will become lifelong memories. If you search
for meaning in these stories, they will be powerful and positive lessons for
you: the patient whom you couldn't save, but who touched a chord deep
within you when he thanked you for being gentle; the family member who
displayed such selflessness when her second child was diagnosed with a
life-threatening disease; the clinician who uttered just a simple word or two
to his colleague, somehow making everything seem manageable and okay.

Such generosity and generativity are characteristic traits of good
leaders. Development of positive leadership strategies is yet another

resilience strategy that will help to empower your practice. Moreover, leadership isn't restricted to those who hold legitimate authority. Recall Sister Dorothea in the previous chapter by Linda Shields. Dot was just ready to give out cups of tea to tired nurses as she was to fight robustly for a cause in management meetings. And remember Maria Stromberger, the nurse who demonstrated incredible courage during World War II.

Leadership is a quality available to all. Now that you have finished this book, you have the knowledge and strategies to become a resilient, empowered nurse. Whether you use what we have presented will help to determine which of the three options you will choose when confronted with a similar situation. We hope you choose the third option and apply the knowledge you have gained in this book in your future practice. That is, you are able to call to mind effective leaders, integrate their qualities into your own practice, and ultimately become the kind of nurse who will support, listen, understand, and inspire others. In the not-too-distant future, you may be the team leader who greets new graduates on their very first day. By enjoying the challenge of helping them grow, you will embody the image of the empowered nurse that was the vision and hope behind this book. We wish you the very best in your nursing career—as an empowered individual, it is yours to create!

REFERENCES

American Association of Colleges of Nursing. (2009). *Nursing shortage fact sheet.* Retrieved from http://www.aacn.nche.edu/media/FactSheets/Nursing Shortage.htm

Australian Safety and Compensation Council. (2007). *Compendium of workers' compensation statistics 2004–05*, Part E, Feature Article: The mechanism - mental stress. Canberra, Australia: Commonwealth of Australia (Department of Employment and Workplace Relations).

Freire, P. (1972). *Pedagogy of the oppressed.* Harmondsworth, England: Penguin.

National Nursing and Nursing Education Taskforce. (2005). Myth: People "drop out" of nursing more than other careers. *Myth busters.* Retrieved from http://www.nhwt.gov.au/documents/N3ET/mythbusters_attrition.pdf

Peterson, C. L. (2007). Work-related stress in Australia. In C. Uyeda (Ed.), *Australian master OHS and environment guide* (2nd ed., pp. 319–335). Sydney, Australia: CCH Publishers.

Regan, A., Howard, R. A., & Oyebode, J. R. (2009). Emotional exhaustion and defense mechanisms in intensive therapy unit nurses. *The Journal of Nervous and Mental Disease, 197*(5), 330–336.

Index

A

Adams, Hunter, 123
Adults, resilience, 8-9
Allanach, B., 48
Anaesthetists, 66
Angelou, Maya, 123
Anorexia, 31-33, 38-39
Antonovsky, Aaron, 8, 133
Anxiety, 138
Appraisals, judgements, 68-70
Aquilino, Mary, 170
Aron, A. P., 64
Askelson, Natoshia, 170
Assertiveness, 83-84
Attitude-behaviour consistency, 87
Auschwitz, 155
Australian College of Children and Young People's Nurses, 157-158, 160
Australian Safety and Compensation Council, 168

B

Bandura, A., 44, 48
Blauner, R., 107
Bonaparte, Napoleon, 162
Brannan, Jane, 171
Buddhism, 140

Buikstra, E., 12
Byron, G. G., 149

C

Caesar, Julius, 162
Calhoun, L. G., 139, 141
Campo, Shelly, 170
Canadian Nurses Association, 50
Case studies. *See* Nursing scenarios
CBT. *See* Cognitive Behavioural Therapy
Centring, 119
Charney, D.S., 15
Children of parents with mental illness (COPMI), 24
Children, resilience, 6-7, 7f
Christ, Jesus, 162
Christianity, 140
Churchill, Winston, 162
Clauss-Ehlers, C., 12
Cognitive Behavioural Therapy (CBT), 13
Colleagues, support bridges, 117-118
Communication, effective
    addressing challenges, 85-86
    audience behaviour, 76-78, 81
    challenges to, 79-81
    example scenario, 75-76

Communication, effective *(cont.)*
  importance of, 79
  introduction to, 75
  key points, 87–88
  persuasion, 86–87
  strategies for, 81–87
Compassion, 83, 161–162
Consequentialism, 34
Convincing communication. *See*
  Communication, effective
Coping skills, 9–10, 167–168. *See also*
  Stressful situations
COPMI. *See* Children of parents with
  mental illness
Courage, 159
Credibility, 82
Crises, coping in. *See* Trauma
Critical incident, 136

D
De Chesnay, Mary, 171
De Pree, M., 23
Deontology, 34
Depression, 138
Difference, tolerance/celebration,
  161
Doctor-nurse game, 93–94
Door-in-the-face strategy, 86
Dutton, D. G., 64

E
Edenborough, M., 14
Eley, R., 12
Emotional responses, 84, 142
Empathy, 83
Epictetus, 91
Estefan, Andrew, 169
Ethical theories, 33–34

Ethics, morals. *See* Nursing practice,
  morals/ethics
Example scenarios. *See* Nursing
  scenarios
Exercise, 124–126, 126*t*
Explanatory styles. *See* Reactive
  styles
External attribution, 62

F
Face needs, 82–83
Family, support bridges, 118–119
Firtko, A., 14
Florence Nightingale Museum, 27
Folkman, S., 125
Foot-in-the-door strategy, 86
Foster, K., 99
Frankl, Viktor, 8–9, 140
Freire, P., 169
Freud, Sigmund, 123
Friends, support bridges, 118
Fromm, E., 107
Functional impacts, reactive styles,
  61–63

G
Gallows humour, 123
Gates, Bill, 161
Gather Together in My Name
  (Angelou), 123
Generation Y characteristics,
  3, 4*t*
Generativity, 17–18
Geocaching, 126
Ghandi, Mahatma, 162
Gilligan, C., 37
Goffman, E., 98
Greef, A., 9–10

Gretter, Lystra, 27
Growth, 139-143. *See also* Posttrau-
    matic growth (PTG)

H

Handbook of Posttraumatic Growth
    (Calhoun, Tedeschi), 141
Happiness, pleasure, 34-35
Hart, Patricia, 171
Hawke, Bob, 157
Health care environment. *See also*
    Workplace adversity
    challenges to communication, 79-81
    characteristics, 3, 4*t*
    workplace adversity, 106-107
Health professions, resilience, 14
Healthcare professionals. *See* Nurses,
    nursing
Heggen, K., 12
Hegney, D., 12
Henderson, A., 159
Holmes, C., 3
Holzhauser, K., 159
Homer, 149
Horizontal violence, 168-169
Human, B., 9-10
Humility, 162
Humour, 123-124

I

Internal attribution, 62-63
International Council of Nurses (ICN),
    150

J

Jackson, D., 14, 108
Jackson, Debra, 171

Jefferson, Thomas, 162
Journal of Clinical Nursing,
    150, 159
Judgements, appraisals, 68-70
Jung, C. G., 137

K

Katsikitis, Mary, 170
Keating, Paul, 151
Kouzes, J., 27

L

Lao-Tzu, 149
Laughter, 123-124
Lazarus, R. S., 125
Leadership
    compassion, 161-162
    courage, 159
    humility, 162
    importance of, 28, 162-163,
        171-172
    introduction to, 149-150
    mistakes, 161
    notable leaders, 23-28, 150-158
    research on, 158-162
    risk taking, 160
    tolerance of difference, 161
    toughness, 160-161
Levi, L., 12
Levi, Primo, 8-9
Listening, 81
Logotherapy, 140
Lothe, E., 12

M

Mandela, Nelson, 162
Mater Hospital, 151-152

McAllister, M., 99
McAndrew, Sue, 170
McCarthy, Emma Maud, 153–155,
    153*f,* 160
McDonald, Glenda, 171
McPhee, Maura, 170
Meditation, 119–120
Mentoring, 109–110
Miasma theory, 25
Mistakes, 161
Morals, ethics. *See* Nursing practice,
    morals/ethics
Music, 122–123

N
Neutral settings, 85
Nietzsche, Friedrich, 140
Nightingale, Florence, 23–28,
    24*f,* 122
Nightingale pledge, 27
Nobel Prize, 150–151
Nonverbal communication, 85
Notes on Nursing (Nightingale), 27
Nurses, communication. *See*
    Communication, effective
Nurses, leadership. *See* Leadership
Nurses, nursing
    becoming effective, 47–48
    compensation, 168
    coping with stress, 117–127
    doctor-nurse game, 93–94
    expectations of, 3
    horizontal violence, 168–169
    making a difference, 39–40
Nurses, nursing *(cont.)*
    resilience, 14–17, 99–100
    retention rates, 167
    strength in, 28
Nurses, team-work. *See* Team-work

Nursing practice, morals/ethics
    example scenario, 31–33, 38–39
    importance of, 40
    introduction to, 31
    making a difference, 39–40
    principles, 33–35
    relational ethics, 36–37
    repositioning, 35–36
    solution focus, 37–39
Nursing scenarios
    coping with stress, 115–116,
        127–128
    effective communication, 75–76
    learning from role models,
        43–44
    morals, ethics, 31–33, 38–39
    resilience, 1–3
    stressful situations, 59–61
    team-work, 92–93, 95–97
    trauma, 135
    workplace stress, 105–106

O
Oberle, K., 35
O'Brien, L., 99
Optimistic explanatory style,
    61–62

P
Paediatric nursing, 157
Parker, V., 12
Patch Adams, 123
Persuasive communication. *See*
    Communication, effective
Pessimistic explanatory style, 63
Pets, 121
Physiological arousal, 64–67
Plank, A., 12

Pleasure, happiness, 34–35
Plumb, Charlie, 9
Positive reinforcement, 86–87
Posner, B., 27
Posttraumatic growth (PTG)
  research, 9, 14
  role models, 18
  trauma, 134, 139–143
Posttraumatic stress disorder (PTSD),
  134, 138
Power structures, 80, 82, 94
Pratt, Jan, 157–159
Preceptor competencies, 50, 51*t*
*The Presentation of Self in Everyday
  Life* (Goffman), 98
Professional support networks, 108–111,
  171
Ptacek, J., 9
PTG. *See* Posttraumatic growth
PTSD. *See* Posttraumatic stress
  disorder

Q

Queen Alexandra's Imperial Military
  Nursing Service (QAIMNS),
  154

R

Raffin-Bouchal, S., 35
Reactive styles
  appraisals, judgements, 68–70
  evaluating, moderating, 63–64,
    167–168
  functional impact, 61–63
  learning to change, 64–70
  physiological arousal, 64–67
Reciprocity, 87
Recognition, trauma, 137–138

Relational ethics, 36–37, 39
Relationship dynamics. *See*
  Team-work
Resilience
  across cultures, communities, 12
  in adults, 8–9
  in children, 6–7
  context-specific skills, 10–11
  coping skills, 9–10
  defining, 6
  developing a store of, 99–100
  dynamic framework of, 11*f*
  example scenario, 1–3
  features of, 11*t*
  health professions, 14
  leadership, 28
  learning, 15, 16*t*
  relevance of, 15–18
  research into, 6–17
  self-efficacy, 98
  stress, 3–17
  at work, 12–13
  workplace adversity, 108
Rickety bridge test, 64–65
Risk taking, 160
Role models. *See also* Leadership
  effective nurses, 47–48
  effective role modelling, 48–51
  example scenario, 43–44
  importance of, 54, 170
  peer, 53–54
  reality shock, 45–46
  self-efficacy, 48
  social learning, 44–45
  where to find, 51–53

S

Salutogenesis, 8
Scenarios. *See* Nursing scenarios

Seacole, Mary, 23, 25-28, 26*f*
Segal, J., 9
Self-efficacy, 48, 91, 96-99
Self-esteem, 91, 96-99
Seligman, M., 15
Shakespeare-Finch, Jane, 171
Sharman, Rachael, 170
Sheehan, Mary Dorothea, 151-153,
    161-162, 172
Shields, Linda, 172
Siebert, Al, 10
Skinner, B. F., 86
Smith, D., 8
Smith, R., 9
Smith, William, 23
Smoll, F., 9
Social learning, 44-45
Solution focus, 37-39
Spirituality, 120
Splitting, 96-97
Stein, L. I., 93-94
Storytelling, 38-39, 169
Stress. *See also* Trauma
    resilience, 3-17
    sources of, 3-5, 168
    workplace adversity, 105-107
Stress, coping with
    example scenario, 115-116,
        127-128
    exercise, 124-126
    humour, laughter, 123-124
    importance of, 128
    introduction to, 115
    managing tips, 18
    meditation, 119-120
    music, 122-123
    in nursing, 117-127
    pets, 121
    relaxing activities, 127
    spirituality, 120

support bridges, 117-119
    volunteerism, 121-122
Stress diathesis model, 5-6, 5*f*
Stressful situations. *See also* Reactive
        styles
    appraisals, judgements, 68-70
    example scenario, 59-61
    introduction to, 59
    physiological arousal, 64-67
    reacting to, 167-168
Stromberger, Maria, 155-157, 156*f*,
    160-161, 172
Styles, Margretta, 150
Support bridges, 117-119
Support networks, 108-111, 171

T
Team-work
    developing resilience, 99-100
    example scenario, 92-93, 95-97
    importance of, 100-101, 170-171
    introduction to, 91-92
    layered scenario, 95-97
    sense of self, 98-99
    team games, 93-95
Tedeschi, R. G., 139, 141
Telstra, 13
Thatcher, Margaret, 162
Thinking clearly. *See* Reactive styles;
        Stressful situations
Toughness, 160-161
Trauma
    defined, 134-135
    example scenario, 135
    growing after, 141-143
    introduction to, 133-134
    outcomes after, 138-143
    subjective nature of, 135-138
    vicarious, 134

U
Utilitarianism, 34

V
Vicarious trauma, 134
Virtue ethics, 35
Volunteerism, 121-122

W
Walker, C., 10
Warne, Tony, 170
Watson, Roger, 150-151, 150*f,* 159

Welch, V., 122
Wiesel, Elie, 8
Wilkes, Lesley, 171
Winch, S., 159
*Wonderful Adventures of Mrs.
    Seacole in Many Lands*
    (Seacole), 27
Workplace adversity
    defined, 106-107
    example scenario, 105-106
    introduction to, 105
    large organisations, 107
    resilience, 108
    support networks, 108-111

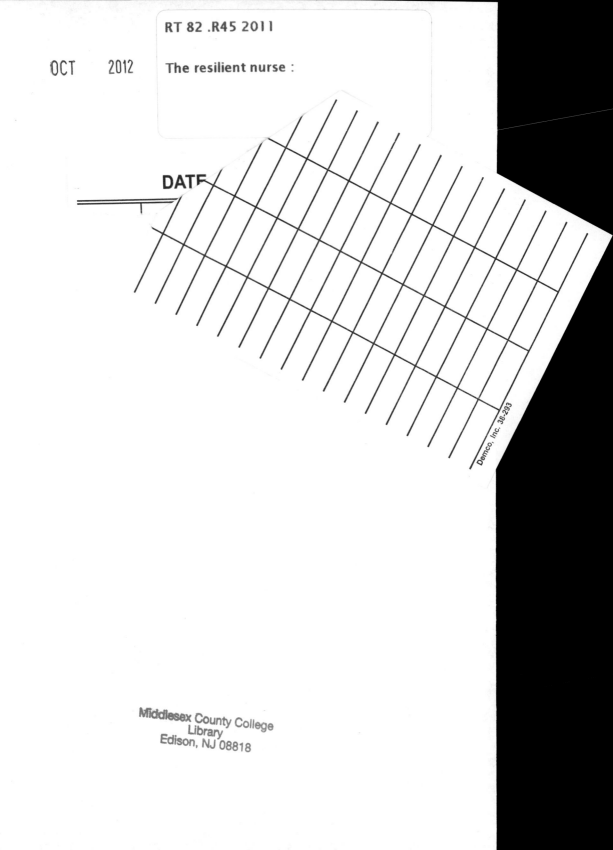